Creation of New Race-Ethnicity Codes and Socioeconomic Status (SES) Indicators for Medicare Beneficiaries

Final Report

Prepared for:
Agency for Healthcare Research and Quality
540 Gather Road
Rockville, MD 20850
Linda G. Greenberg, Ph.D.
Federal Project Officer

and

Centers for Medicare & Medicaid Services
7500 Security Boulevard
Baltimore, MD 21244-1850
Barbara Crawley, MS
Elizabeth Goldstein, Ph.D.
Federal Project Officers

CMS Contract Number: 500-00-0024, Task No. 21

Prepared by:
RTI International
Research Triangle Park, NC

Investigators
Arthur J. Bonito, Ph.D.
Carla Bann, Ph.D.
Celia Eicheldinger, M.S.
Lisa Carpenter, B.S.

January 2008

This project was funded by the Centers for Medicare & Medicaid Services through an interagency agreement with the Agency for Healthcare Research and Quality under contract no. 500-00-0024, Task No. 21.

This final report was submitted in July 2006.

The statements contained in this report are solely those of the authors and do not necessarily reflect the views or policies of the Centers for Medicare & Medicaid Services or the Agency for Healthcare Research and Quality. RTI assumes responsibility for the accuracy and completeness of the information contained in this report.

Acknowledgments

We want to acknowledge the contributions to the work performed in this report of our programmer Ann Larsen; our primary word processor for the tabular appendices, Joyce Clay-Brooks; Loraine Monroe the word processor for the final report; and our technical editor, Marceline Murawski. Without their special skills, commitment, and hard work, this report would not have been completed on time. We also want to acknowledge the helpful comments, interest, and support of Barbara Crawley, the primary Centers for Medicare and Medicaid Services (CMS) Project Officer.

Table of Contents

LIST OF TABLES

FIGURE

APPENDIXES

The following appendixes can be obtained by contacting Dr. Ernest Moy, Medical Officer Center for Quality Improvement and Patient Safety, Agency for Healthcare Research and Quality. Email: ernest.moy@ahrq.hhs.gov.

A.   Additional Tabulations and Statistical Testing During the Validation of the Socioeconomic Status Index

B.   Cancer Screening Tables

C.   Diabetes Prevention Tables

D.   Ambulatory Care Sensitive Condition Tables

E.   Common Hospital Diagnosis Tables

F.   Documentation of the Medicare Claims Data Presented in the Tables

G.   Codebook for the Analytic File

H.   Tables of Denominators for Weighted and Unweighted National and MSA Tabulations (Bound Separately)

I.   SUDAAN® Output for the Multivariate Analysis

Creation of New Race and Socioeconomic Status Indicators for Medicare Beneficiaries (Sub-Task 2)

EXECUTIVE SUMMARY

Objectives

This project sub-task is a continuation of an earlier task order project (Contract Number 500-00-0024, Task 8) *Health Disparities: Measuring Health Care Use and Access for Racial/Ethnic Populations* (2005) intended to identify race/ethnic disparities in the use of selected Medicare covered services. This sub-task has two objectives. The first is to create and validate an acceptable measure of socioeconomic status (SES) that could be incorporated into further analyses of health care disparities among the racial/ethnic groups participating in the Medicare program. The second objective is to prepare tabulations (using an improved race/ethnicity measure created in the earlier project) that incorporate the SES variable (as well as age and gender) in such a way, that differences in utilization associated with race/ethnicity are highlighted while the effects of the aforementioned covariates are controlled or held constant.

To rigorously investigate whether there are racial/ethnic health care disparities present in Medicare, it is critical to be able to assess the extent to which disparities are associated with an improved race/ethnicity variable alone, rather than with socioeconomic status (SES), because the impacts of these variables are often confounded. Thus we sought to examine apparent racial/ethnic health care disparities while other important factors, such as SES, age, and gender were controlled. In the past, it has not been possible to do this kind of analysis using Medicare administrative data alone because the enrollment database (EDB) which contains the person-level characteristics of beneficiaries does not include an appropriate variable or surrogate to measure SES. In this sub-task we created and validated such a measure, building on our efforts in the earlier project to geocode beneficiaries' addresses and link them to US Census data on their block group. In addition, accuracy of the race/ethnicity coding on the EDB was increased by using the improved race/ethnicity measure we developed in the earlier project. Because the current task was based largely on our previous efforts, it is important to understand the work done in the earlier project to lay the foundation for the work performed in this task. For that reason, a summary of this previous work has been included.

Research Methods

Race/Ethnicity Coding on the EDB. The race data on the EDB has historically been obtained from the Social Security Administration's (SSA's) master beneficiary record (MBR). Until 1980, applicants filing for a Social Security number completed a form SS-5. The race item only permitted classification of race as "White", "Black", or "Other", and missing responses were coded as "Unknown". In 1980, the SSA's race categories were expanded to "Hispanic"; (non-Hispanic) "White"; (non-Hispanic) "Black"; Asian, Asian-American, or Pacific Islander; American Indian or Alaska Native; and "Unknown". When the SSA began enrolling applicants at birth by extracting data from birth certificates, it was not considered necessary to include race

1

or ethnicity (Scott, 1999). In 1994, the expanded race/ethnicity codes from the SS-5 form were incorporated into the Medicare EDB. This update was repeated in 1997 and 2000, and annually since then. In 1997, the Health Care Financing Administration (now the centers for Medicare & Medicaid Services, or CMS) conducted a post card survey to improve the EDB's race/ethnicity coding. Following these efforts, researchers assessed the improvement in the EDB's race/ethnicity data, and concluded that while there was a noticeable improvement in the coding, identification of Hispanics, Asians/Pacific Islanders, and American Indians/Alaska Natives was still incomplete (Arday, et al 2000; Eggers and Greenberg, 2000; and Waldo, 2005).

Assessing Current Status of EDB Race/Ethnicity. The first step in our earlier project was to assess the correctness of the EDB race/ethnicity coding on the mid-2003 EDB. To do this, we compared the race/ethnicity on the EDB for the almost 831,000 respondents to the 2000-2002 Medicare CAHPS surveys (also known as the Medicare Satisfaction Surveys). The survey self-response to the race/ethnicity items served as the gold standard against which the accuracy of the EDB race/ethnicity codes was assessed. We used sensitivity, specificity, positive predictive value, negative predictive value, and Kappa to measure agreement between the two sources of race/ethnicity data. The accuracy of the EDB was highest for non-Hispanic Blacks, with all measures above 90 percent. Non-Hispanic Whites were the next most accurately coded on the EDB. Only specificity (62 percent) and Kappa (0.71) were less than 90 percent for non-Hispanic Whites. The moderate level of specificity and Kappa reflect a considerable number of self-reported non-White CAHPS respondents coded as White on the EDB. Sensitivity for American Indians/Alaska Natives was only 36 percent and the positive predictive value just 60 percent, contributing to a low Kappa (0.45).

Hispanics and Asians/Pacific Islanders were the minority groups of particular interest since we planned to develop an algorithm based on their unique surnames to improve their coding on the EDB. The sensitivity for Hispanic coding on the EDB was a low 30 percent and for Asia/Pacific Islander it was 55 percent. Closer examination revealed that these low sensitivities largely reflected self-identified Hispanics coded as White on the EDB, and self-identified Asians coded as Other on the EDB. The Kappas were 0.45 and 0.66 respectively for Hispanic and Asian/Pacific Islander Medicare beneficiaries, reflecting the low sensitivities, but the other measures were acceptable at approximately 90 percent or more.

Developing an Algorithm to Accurately Impute Race/Ethnicity. Having established the need to improve coding for the Hispanic and Asian/Pacific Islander Medicare beneficiaries we undertook creation of imputation algorithms for both minority groups. The algorithms made use of information on the EDB, such language preference for mailing informational materials, source of their race/ethnicity code, and whether they resided in Hawaii or Puerto Rico. The algorithms also used Hispanic (Word and Perkins, 1996) and Asian/Pacific Islander (Falkenstein and Word, 2002) surname lists developed by the U.S. Census Bureau. The Hispanic surname list included a percentage for each name representing the proportion of times a household headed by an individual with a particular Hispanic surname was indeed in an Hispanic household as reported to the Census. There were similar percentages for the Asian/Pacific Islander surnames. We also considered typical Hispanic and Asian first names.

We incorporated these pieces of information into a SAS program that, through an iterative process which differed slightly for Hispanics and Asians/Pacific Islanders, created an algorithm that improved the race/ethnicity variable. In the algorithm, a beneficiary was considered Hispanic (or Asian): if the beneficiary's surname was identified as Hispanic (Asian) by the Census at least 70 percent of the time, otherwise, if the EDB coded the beneficiary as Hispanic (Asian), otherwise, if the person was a resident of Puerto Rico (Hawaii), otherwise, if the beneficiary preferred to get program information in Spanish, otherwise, if the beneficiary's first name had Hispanic (Asian) origins, and the surname was considered Hispanic (Asian) at least 50 percent of the time by the Census. Conditions were also identified under which a race/ethnicity changed according to these rules was restored to its EDB code.

Assessment of the Algorithm. Using the self-reported race/ethnicity data from the 2000-2002 Medicare CAHPS survey respondents as the gold standard again, we assessed the results of applying the algorithm to the CAHPS respondents. We found the algorithm significantly improved the race/ethnicity categorization of Hispanic and Asian/Pacific Islander Medicare beneficiaries. Among Hispanic beneficiaries, sensitivity improved from 30 to 77 percent, the Kappa coefficient rose from 0.43 to 0.79, and the other measures (specificity and predictive values) remained virtually unchanged. The improvement for Asian/Pacific Islander beneficiaries was equally impressive – sensitivity rose from 55 to 80 percent, Kappa increased from 0.66 to 0.80, and the other measures were not materially changed. Applying the algorithm to the entire 41.7 million persons on the mid-2003 EDB resulted in changing race/ethnicity codes to Hispanic for nearly two million Medicare beneficiaries and to Asian/Pacific Islander for three hundred thousand beneficiaries. Hispanics increased from 2.2 percent of Medicare beneficiaries to 7.0 percent, and Asians/Pacific Islanders increased from 1.4 percent to 2.0 percent.

Geocoding Beneficiary Addresses. As part of the earlier project, we employed a software package from GeoLytics, Incorporated called Geocode CD (release 2.60) to geocode the addresses of Medicare beneficiaries listed on the mid-2003 EDB. Because using GeoCode CD required the elements of beneficiary addresses in a very particular order, we needed to clean and reorder the addresses before processing them. The process of geocoding was performed to generate a FIPS code that would allow linkage of beneficiaries to the socioeconomic characteristics of their residential neighborhood (block group) from the 2000 Census. We were able to run 87.5 percent of the 41.7 million Medicare beneficiary's addresses though the geocoding process. Those that were not processed either had a box or route number and no street address or were foreign addresses, conditions that Geocode CD could not handle. We obtained FIPS codes for 99.2 percent of those processed by invoking options that allowed the use of variations from the input address when that address could not be found in the Geocode CD database.

Creating an SES Index. In the current sub-task, we used the beneficiary-linked block group data to develop a single measure of SES for beneficiaries that incorporated the common strains of the separate socioeconomic variables of their neighborhood (block group) extracted from the Census. Following the work of Krieger et al. (2003a) at Harvard University, we used the same block group level socioeconomic characteristics she extracted from the Census to create an SES index for the sample of 1.96 million Medicare beneficiaries selected for study in our previous task order project. These characteristics were representative of the occupational, income, wealth, and educational characteristics of residents in the block group.

Just as Krieger et al (2003a) did, we performed a principal components analysis of the following seven Census variables: percentage of persons in the labor force who are unemployed; percentage of persons living below poverty level; median household income; median value of owner-occupied dwellings; percentage of persons 25 years of age or older with less than a 12th grade education; the percentage of persons 25 years of age or older completing four or more years of college; and the percentage of households that average one or more persons per room. The weights from the first principal component were used to create an SES index score for the 1.57 million beneficiaries in the Medicare sample who had a FIPS code and block group Census data associated with their address. The continuous range of SES index scores was standardized so scores could range between 0 and 100. The scores were then grouped into four categories to facilitate tabular analysis.

Validating the SES Index. Before using the four category SES measure in tabulations we validated it. We used the national probability sample of Medicare beneficiary respondents to the three Medicare fee-for-service CAHPS surveys for 2002-2004 as the basis for our validation. In addition to the CAHPS survey measures, we had requested and received some income-related information for CAHPS respondents from the Social Security Administration (SSA)-- the indexed monthly earnings (IME) that were taxed for Social Security purposes while the beneficiary was paying the Social Security tax, and the monthly benefit amount (MBA) that Social Security is currently paying beneficiaries.

The first step in the validation process involved computing the SES index scores for the full validation sample of over 381,000 Medicare fee-for-service CAHPS respondents and creating the four category SES measure. We next computed the means of the two SSA variables within each level of SES and we also cross tabulated the two SSA variables with SES scores. We found that the mean IMEs increased significantly as the SES level rose. The distribution of beneficiaries across the four categories of SES according to the four categories of their IME was also highly significant, indicating that, proportionately more beneficiaries with lower IME were classified in lower SES categories, and proportionately more of those with higher IME were classified in higher SES categories. We also found that the mean MBA increased significantly as the SES category went from the lowest to the highest. The cross tabulation of MBA and SES showed a similar significant association, with proportionately more low MBA beneficiaries in the lowest SES category and proportionately more high MBA beneficiaries in the highest SES category.

In addition to the two SSA variables, we had several others from the CAHPS survey -- having additional insurance (not including Medicaid), having private insurance to cover prescription drugs, reporting health status to be fair or poor, and achieving educational status no higher than high school graduate -- and one from the EDB -- whether or not a beneficiary is simultaneously eligible for both Medicare and Medicaid -- that we believed should be related to SES. Eligibility for both Medicare and Medicaid was significantly associated with SES: eligibility was greatest among the lowest SES category. The associations between the four CAHPS measures and the SES variable were also highly significant. The direction of the associations was as expected: larger percentages of persons in poor or fair health and persons who had no more than a high school education were in the lower SES categories, and fewer persons with other insurance (not including Medicaid) and private prescription drug coverage were in the lower SES categories.

Analysis

Sample Selection. The analyses planned for this sub-task were performed on a probability sample of 1.96 million Medicare beneficiaries selected for analysis in the previous task order contract and reported on in the report titled *Health Disparities: Measuring Health Care Use and Access for Racial/Ethnic Populations* (2005). This sample was selected from the full 10 segments of the mid-2003 unloaded EDB. To be eligible for inclusion in the sample, beneficiaries must have been enrolled in traditional fee-for-service (FFS) Medicare (Part A, Part B, or both) for the full 12 months of the 2002 calendar year and not have been enrolled in a Group Health Organization at all during that calendar year. In addition, beneficiaries must have been alive for the full 12 months of calendar year 2002. We set these criteria to allow the maximum opportunity (period of time) for beneficiaries to submit claims documenting their use of preventive and other Medicare covered services.

The primary sampling goal at the time this sample was selected was to have sufficient sample size to provide equally precise estimates of health care utilization for the different racial/ethnic groups. We therefore sampled such that, to the extent possible, the same number of Medicare beneficiaries would be included in the sample in each of the different racial/ethnic groups. The sampling rates based on the NEWRACE code was 11 percent for Black Medicare beneficiaries, 1.2 percent for White, 26 percent for Hispanic, 71 percent for Asian/Pacific Islander, and 100 percent of American Indian/Alaska Native, Other, and Unknown.

Tabulations. We redesigned a number of tabulations performed for the earlier CMS task order to identify health care disparities among Medicare beneficiaries by race/ethnicity. The tabulations for this project incorporated a four categorical version of the SES index score along with race/ethnicity, gender (where appropriate) and age group. The health care utilization variables analyzed in the tabulations included the use of cancer screening services, services for the secondary prevention of complications of diabetes, hospitalizations for ambulatory sensitive conditions that are indicators of inadequate primary care, and the number, length, and expenditures for common hospitalizations experienced by Medicare beneficiaries. These were extracted for the sample members from their 2002 Medicare claims.

As part of the expansion of the tabulations to include SES, the tabulations were done for the nation as a whole and repeated for the 10 metropolitan statistical areas (MSAs) where the largest number of Hispanics and Asians/Pacific Islanders 65 years of age and older reside. Since four of the MSAs were in common between the two groups of ten MSAs, the tabulations were only prepared for the nation as a whole and the 16 unique MSAs.

Multivariate Modeling. In an effort to better understand the overall impact of the SES measure on the disparities in health care utilization between White Medicare beneficiaries and those who are members of racial/ethnic minorities at the national level, we estimated several multivariate logistic regression analytic models. Our analytic approach involved three steps. The first was to estimate the size of the White-minority group differences in utilization, controlling only on gender and age group, and then we re-estimated the differences by controlling on SES as well as gender and age group in the model. In the final step, we re-estimated the differences in utilization controlling on the interaction between SES and race/ethnicity as well as gender and age group.

We conducted regression model analyses on seven of the 45 utilization measures included in the tabulations, and only at the national level. They included three cancer screening measures (past 12 month receipt of: the combination of mammogram and Pap smear for women, the prostate specific antigen (PSA) test for men, and any of the three colorectal cancer screening tests for both sexes), three diabetes secondary preventive services for beneficiaries identified as diagnosed with diabetes (past 12 month receipt of: physiologic testing (hemoglobin A1c, lipid profile, or micro albumin) to monitor insulin needs, an eye exam, and instruction in self-care (diabetes education and self-monitoring)), and whether or not a beneficiary had a hospital or emergency department admission with a diagnosis of any of 15 ambulatory care sensitive conditions (ACSCs) we included.

For the first six service use measures, minorities typically had lower utilization than Whites while equal or higher would have been better. For the ACSC measure, the difference in utilization was reversed because a higher level of hospitalization for these diagnoses is poorer quality care considered largely avoidable with appropriate and timely ambulatory care. Furthermore, the magnitude of disparities between minority beneficiaries and Whites represented by these seven utilization measures ranged from very small or none to very large or substantial.

The regression models confirmed that controlling the impact of SES (as well as age and gender) typically reduces the size of the utilization difference between Whites and minorities, i.e. the disparity. The amount of the reduction varied with the measure of use and the minority, however, it is important to note that it never came close to eliminating the difference. A final set of regression models was run to investigate whether there is a statistical interaction between race/ethnicity and SES that impacts the differences in utilization. We found that there were interactions, and that the reduction in differences between Whites and minorities varied according to race/ethnicity and level of SES. The interaction between race/ethnicity and SES revealed that the differences between Whites and minorities were not uniform across SES levels, but were often larger among beneficiaries in the higher SES levels than they were in the lower SES levels. Based on so few measures of utilization, however, these results are suggestive at best, and indicate that analyses of additional utilization variables are needed.

Conclusions

Important Results. Both of the objectives of this sub-task were achieved. We developed an index of socioeconomic status (SES) for a probability sample of nearly 1.6 million Medicare beneficiaries stratified by an upgraded measure of race/ethnicity. Development of the upgraded race/ethnicity was itself an achievement because it made it possible to more confidently examine racial/ethnic disparities with regard to the health care utilization of Black, Hispanic and Asian/Pacific Islander Medicare beneficiaries.

We developed the SES index from Census data representing the beneficiaries' residential neighborhood. The methods we employed were similar to those of other researchers seeking to measure the impact of socioeconomic status on disparities in health services utilization. The resulting SES measure was subsequently validated on a large independent sample of Medicare beneficiaries using economic, social, and behavioral measures presumed to be related to SES that we obtained from the Social Security Administration and CMS (data from the EDB and fee-for-service CAHPS). The validation activity showed that these variables were moderately related to the SES measure and in the expected direction, exactly what one wants in the validation of an index based on multiple related items. The associations were all very highly statistically significant.

We also achieved the second objective which was to generate tabulations on a variety of health services utilization measures controlling on SES, as well as age and gender, to provide a better estimate of potential disparities between Whites and minority group members in their use of health care. While limited time and resources prevented analysis of the hundreds of tabulations prepared, the results of our limited multivariate modeling analyses confirmed that controlling on SES did reduce the difference in health care utilization between White and minority Medicare beneficiaries. Our examination of the interaction between race/ethnicity and SES indicated that these differences in utilization were often smaller among beneficiaries in the lower SES categories than in the higher ones.

Limitations. As we have indicated, the results of this sub-task utilizing the SES index are an important contribution to the understanding of racial/ethnic disparities in the use of health care. The results of the race/ethnicity imputation algorithm used in this sub-task also represents an important expansion in the use of a large and potentially fruitful administrative database that to date has been of limited use for examining disparities beyond White and Black differences. There are limitations to the work and aspects of it for which additional research is needed.

While the naming algorithm did greatly improve the coding of Hispanics and Asians/Pacific Islanders, there is still room for further improvement, not to mention the need for continual updating as new beneficiaries are added to the Medicare program. We did nothing to improve the accuracy of the American Indian/Alaska Native group and our analysis suggests that they remain seriously under-identified. There may be some way to better identify who these beneficiaries are through reservation addresses or sources of care used. This should be further investigated as the available data show this group to be particularly vulnerable to not using health care as much as others.

The geocoding of beneficiary addresses has allowed researchers to associate some type of SES measures based on place of residence with most Medicare beneficiaries, but not all. Because many of the addresses were box numbers, rural route, in Puerto Rico or a foreign country and could not be geocoded by the software, they were not linked to the Census data needed to create the SES index. Further research should be undertaken to determine how these addresses should be handled.

Further, preliminary examination of a sample of geocoded addresses indicates that employing some of the Geocode CD software's options may have resulted in misidentifying a small proportion of block groups. In the future it would be advisable to more thoroughly investigate the impact of this misidentification on results.

Finally, our multivariate analysis and the associated tabulations were produced using available Medicare claims data from 2002, and may not represent the situation in 2006. Just as the race/ethnicity algorithm and geocoding process should be updated, so also should the 2002 sample and claims data, to reflect the new beneficiaries in Medicare and any improvements made in the more equitable receipt of care.

Creation of New Race-Ethnicity Codes and Socioeconomic Status (SES) Indicators for Medicare Beneficiaries

Final Report, Sub-Task 2

1. INTRODUCTION

1.1   Background

There has been considerable interest during the past decade or so in reducing racial and ethnic disparities in the use of health services. Understanding whether disparities result from sub-cultural differences in the practices of minorities or reflect the impact of different socioeconomic circumstances is key to designing interventions to reduce disparities. Studying racial/ethnic disparities in health care among Medicare beneficiaries should be close to ideal because it largely eliminates insurance- and cost-related access barriers as explanations of health care disparities. To a large extent, differences in access to health care are expected to be minimal for Medicare beneficiaries because there is a standard set of benefits for which all beneficiaries are eligible. In addition, there are assistance programs available to reduce the cost burdens associated with the monthly premiums for Part B (Supplemental Medical Insurance) as well as any coinsurance and deductibles for low income persons.

To rigorously investigate whether and where there are racial/ethnic health care disparities present in Medicare, it is critical to be able to assess the extent to which any disparities are associated with race or ethnicity rather than socioeconomic status (SES), because the impacts of these variables are often confounded, while other important factors such as age and gender are controlled as well. It has not been possible in the past to do this kind of analysis using Medicare administrative data alone because the enrollment database which contains the person-level characteristics of beneficiaries does not include an appropriate variable or surrogate to measure SES.

In addition, analyses of racial/ethnic health care disparities in the Medicare program have been limited to comparisons between White and Black/African American beneficiaries because of problems with the quality and completeness of coding on the EDB for Hispanic and Latino, Asian and Pacific Island, and American Indian and Alaska Native beneficiaries. It has been demonstrated that large numbers of beneficiaries of Hispanic and Asian decent have been erroneously identified on the Medicare enrollment database (EDB) (Arday et al., 2000; Eggers and Greenberg, 2000; Waldo, 2005). In a previous task order project (Contract Number 500-00-0024, Task 8, *Health Disparities: Measuring Health Care Use and Access for Racial/Ethnic Populations,* 2005) to identify racial and ethnic disparities in health care utilization and access among Medicare beneficiaries that RTI conducted for the Centers for Medicare & Medicaid Services (CMS), our first objective was to assess the accuracy of the racial/ethnic coding of beneficiaries listed in the EDB. We confirmed the same incomplete and incorrect coding of race/ethnicity. The second objective of that project was to develop an algorithm making use of surnames and other available information to upgrade the coding of the EDB race/ethnicity variable for Hispanic and Asian/Pacific Islander beneficiaries and to validate the results of the algorithm. We completed that work and a description of it is included in this report because we relied upon it. Some time prior to initiation of our work, CMS had negotiated an interagency agreement with the Indian Health Service to identify American Indian and Alaska Native beneficiaries to Medicare. We used the version of the EDB that included the upgraded American Indian/Alaska Native coding.

In addition to the incomplete and incorrect coding of race/ethnicity on the EDB that would make it difficult to conduct a rigorous assessment of the separate impact of race/ethnicity and SES on the use of health services, as we indicated above, the EDB does not contain any measures or indicators of SES. To remedy this situation, in the previous task order project (Contract Number 500-00-0024, Task 8, *Health Disparities: Measuring Health Care Use and Access for Racial/Ethnic Populations*, 2005), RTI successfully geocoded the addresses of 36.2 million Medicare beneficiaries to obtain a Federal Information Processing Standard (FIPS) code for the US Census Block Group (the smallest US Census area for which there are economic data reported from the Census) in which the beneficiary's address was located. We were then able to associate socioeconomic characteristics of a beneficiary's neighborhood with the beneficiary, although no analysis was done using this census data. The former task order contract under which the original surname algorithm and geocoding work was performed is the foundation on which the current task order project has been conducted.

1.2 Purpose

The work conducted in task two of the current task order contract (contract 500-00-0024, task 21) with the Centers for Medicare & Medicaid Services (CMS) was undertaken with the purpose of further developing the work completed by RTI under the previous task order contract with CMS (contract 500-00-0024, task 8) in the preparation of the 2005 report titled *Health Disparities: Measuring Health Care Use and Access for Racial/Ethnic Populations*. The goal of this work is to empirically specify and isolate the effect of differences in SES from what are presently described as disparities in health care utilization associated with race and ethnicity among Medicare beneficiaries. The race and ethnicity variable developed to improve upon the coding of race/ethnicity available at the time on the Medicare enrollment database (EDB) used in the previous report was again used in this report. A summary of the naming algorithm work performed in the earlier study is presented in the Methods and Data section of this report.

The task activities associated with this work were made possible through an interagency agreement and transfer of funds from the Agency for Healthcare Research and Quality (AHRQ) to CMS. These task activities included the following:

(1) Hold a kickoff meeting, prepare monthly written progress reports, and participate in telephone conference calls as requested;

(2) Develop and validate a measure of SES for Medicare beneficiaries;

(3) Update the existing analytic data file with the new SES variable;

(4) Develop tabular presentations of descriptive statistics on use of selected preventive health services (cancer screening and secondary diabetes prevention), ambulatory sensitive conditions, and average length of stay and expenditures for hospitalizations common to Medicare beneficiaries based on the claims based on a previously selected weighted sample of 1.96 million. Do this for the nation as a whole as well as for designated metropolitan statistical areas (MSAs) – the top 10 for number of elderly Asians and Hispanics separately). This activity will also include limited multivariate logistic regression analyses of selected measures of utilization to summarize the impact of race/ethnicity, SES, age group, and gender.

(5) Prepare a final report describing the work and provide the analytic data file, a codebook for the analytic data file, and copies of the programs used to create the variables in the tabulations.

1.3   Objectives

The objectives of the work performed under the second task in this task order were twofold. First, we wanted to create and validate a composite measure of SES based not on individual-level measures but on variables extracted from the 2000 U.S. Census that have been used to define the SES of beneficiaries' residential neighborhoods (block group). Because we were interested in income-related variables, the smallest aggregate unit for which this kind of data is made available by the Census is the block group, thus our choice of it as the area constituting the beneficiaries' residential neighborhood.

Our second objective in task two was to build upon the set of tabulations created for the previously completed task order discussed above. We were interested in building upon those tabulations in two ways. The first was by including SES in the tabulations along with the improved measure of race/ethnicity (that we created in the previous task order), and age group and gender. The second was to replicate the tabulations done at the national level for the 10 MSAs with the greatest concentration of Asian and Hispanics Medicare beneficiaries. Since the Census does not identify Medicare beneficiaries, we used the number of Asian, Native Hawaiian, and Pacific Islanders age 65 and over, and a similar number for Hispanics and Latinos, as our proxy for identifying the top 10 MSAs for both groups of Medicare beneficiaries.

1.4   Organization of this report

This first section of the report has described the background and purpose of this task order project. The remaining four sections of this report are devoted to descriptions of the work performed and the deliverables prepared. The next section discusses the general methods and data used to accomplish the objectives of the task. Section 3 describes how we developed and validated the SES index that we used in the tabulations. The fourth section describes the tabulations prepared in this task order and presented in separate Appendices. Section 5 discusses the limited multivariate logistic regression analyses performed to begin the onerous task of understanding the association of race/ethnicity, SES, age, and gender on disparities in health care use among Medicare beneficiaries. There are also six appendices to this report. The first and last ones (Appendix A and Appendix F) are included as part of the final report. The other appendices (B through E) are bound separately but are meant to be used in tandem with this report. They have been bound separately for the convenience of persons who may need to work with them in preparing other reports or presentations.

2. METHODS AND DATA[1]

2.1   Improving the Race/Ethnicity Coding of Medicare Beneficiaries

History of EDB Race/Ethnicity Coding. The race/ethnicity code on the Medicare EDB is obtained from the Social Security Administration's (SSA's) master beneficiary record (MBR). From 1935 to 1980, the Social Security application form (SS-5) only allowed classification of a person's race into "White," "Black," or "Other" categories. In addition, "Unknown" was used to classify persons who did not report any race. The codes from the SS-5 were incorporated into the MBR. The number of race/ethnicity categories on the SS-5 form was expanded in 1980 to six: "White (non-Hispanic)"; "Black (non-Hispanic)"; "Hispanic"; "Asian, Asian-American, or Pacific Islander"; "American Indian or Alaska Native"; and "Unknown." In 1989, the SSA began to enroll new participants at birth, extracting data from birth certificates rather than requiring applicants to file form SS-5; however, the race/ethnicity information on the birth certificate was not included in the data extraction because it was considered unnecessary for the administration of the SSA program. Since 1989, the only persons filing an SS-5 form have been those requesting a new number or a name change (Scott, 1999).

In 1994, race data from the SS-5 forms with the expanded race/ethnicity codes were integrated into the Medicare EDB in an effort to correct erroneous codes and fill in missing ones. This action changed the race/ethnicity coding for more than 2.5 million beneficiaries (Lauderdale and Goldberg, 1996). This update using the SS-5 form with the expanded race/ethnicity codes was conducted again in 1997 and 2000, and has been conducted on an annual basis since then. The Medicare program has also been working with the Indian Health Service to improve the coding of American Indians and Alaska Natives.

To correct miscoded data and further reduce the amount of missing race/ethnicity information, in 1997 the Health Care Financing Administration (now the Centers for Medicare & Medicaid Services, or CMS) conducted a postcard survey of nearly 2.2 million beneficiaries. Included in the survey were beneficiaries with: Hispanic surnames, Hispanic countries of birth, or beneficiaries coded "Other" or missing race/ethnicity data. The survey resulted in code changes for approximately 858,000 beneficiaries (Arday et al., 2000). These efforts clearly improved the EDB's race/ethnicity data. Nonetheless, comparisons of the EDB race/ethnicity codes to the self-reported race/ethnicity from the Medicare Current Beneficiary Survey (MCBS) indicated that identification of Hispanics, Asians/Pacific Islanders, and American Indians/Alaska Natives was still incomplete and might result in biased analyses involving these groups (Arday et al., 2000; Eggers and Greenberg, 2000; Waldo, 2005).

Assessment of the Accuracy of Race/Ethnicity Coding on the EDB. The accuracy of the Medicare EDB race/ethnicity code was further assessed by the RTI researchers working on the recently completed Health Disparities project referred to earlier. This assessment consisted

---

[1] The assessment of the EDB race/ethnicity data, creation of the algorithm for imputing Hispanic and Asian/Pacific Islanders, selection of the sample of 1.96 million Medicare fee-for-service beneficiaries, and geocoding of beneficiary addresses discussed in this section was performed by RTI under CMS Contract Number 500-00-0024, Task 8 and has been adapted for this report from the project final report, *Health Disparities: Measuring Health Care Use and Access for Racial/Ethnic Populations* dated April 2005.

of a comparative analysis of the EDB race/ethnicity code with self-reported race/ethnicity data obtained from 830,728 Medicare beneficiary respondents to the 2000-2002 Medicare CAHPS surveys. The analysis investigated the accuracy of the six race/ethnicity classifications used in the EDB race/ethnicity code (non-Hispanic White, non-Hispanic Black, Hispanic, Asian/Pacific Islander, American Indian/Alaska Native, and Unknown/Other). The measures calculated and presented in Table 2.1 to assess the accuracy of the EDB codes include: sensitivity,[2] specificity,[3] positive predictive value[4] (PPV), negative predictive value[5] (NPV), and the Kappa[6] coefficient of inter-rater reliability.

Relative to self-reported data, the accuracy of the EDB was greatest for non-Hispanic Black Medicare beneficiaries: sensitivity was 97.4 percent, specificity was 98.8 percent, PPV was 86.3 percent, NPV was 99.8 percent, and a Kappa coefficient of 0.91 was observed. Non-Hispanic White beneficiaries were the next most accurately identified group on the EDB. Sensitivity was high (99.3 percent), but specificity was just 61.7 percent, suggesting that a sizeable proportion of beneficiaries who were not White were incorrectly coded as White. The PPV and NPV were 91.7 and 95.7 percent, respectively, but the Kappa coefficient was only moderately high at 0.71, reflecting the lower level of specificity. Sensitivity for American Indian/Alaska Native beneficiaries was very low at 35.7 percent, and the PPV was low at 59.9 percent. Specificity and NPV for this group, however, were exceptionally high at 99.9 and 99.7 percent, respectively. The low Kappa coefficient of 0.45 reflects the low sensitivity of the EDB for this group.

---

[2] The percentage of persons who self-reported themselves to be of a particular race/ethnicity who are coded as being of that race on the EDB.

[3] The percentage of persons who self-reported themselves not to be of a particular race/ethnicity who are coded as not being of that race on the EDB.

[4] The percentage of persons coded in a particular race/ethnicity category on the EDB who really were of that race according to their self-report.

[5] The percentage of persons not coded in a particular race/ethnicity category on the EDB who really were not of that race according to their self-report.

[6] Kappa measures agreement between two independent race/ethnicity codes for the same person being coded, in this case between the self-reported and EDB race/ethnicity codes, where a coefficient of 1.00 represents perfect agreement and 0.00 is an absolute lack of agreement.

Table 2.1
Accuracy and agreement between EDBRACE and SELFRACE

| Race/ethnicity | | EDBRACE | | Accuracy and agreement measures for EDBRACE | | | | |
| | | | | | | Positive predictive | Negative predictive | |
SELFRACE		Yes	No	Sensitivity	Specificity	value	value	Kappa
White	Yes	667,573	4,420	99.3%	61.7%	91.7%	95.7%	0.71
	No	60,794	97,941					
Black	Yes	57,867	1,515	97.4	98.8	86.3	99.8	0.91
	No	9,209	762,137					
Hispanic	Yes	12,953	30,974	29.5	99.9	92.7	96.2	0.43
	No	1,025	785,776					
A/PI	Yes	8,008	6,626	54.7	99.8	84.5	99.2	0.66
	No	1,469	814,625					
AI/AN	Yes	1,194	2,150	35.7	99.9	59.9	99.7	0.45
	No	799	826,585					
Other/	Yes	478	27,158	1.7	98.8	4.9	96.7	0.01
Unknown	No	9,357	793,735					

Source: EDBRACE is from the mid-2003 Medicare EDB and SELFRACE is from Medicare CAHPS fee-for-service, managed care enrollee, and disenrollee surveys for 2000-2002. Table taken from the final report for CMS Contract Number 500-00-0024, Task 8 and has been reprinted for this report from the project final report, *Health Disparities: Measuring Health Care Use and Access for Racial/Ethnic Populations* dated April 2005.

The focus of the project, however, was on Hispanic and Asian/Pacific Islander beneficiaries because earlier research had shown that the sensitivity of the EDB was especially low for these groups. Indeed, sensitivity of the EDB for Hispanic beneficiaries was only 29.5 percent, but specificity (99.9 percent), PPV (92.7 percent), and NPV (96.2 percent) were very high. The Kappa agreement coefficient of 0.43 reflected the low level of correct identification of Hispanic beneficiaries on the EDB represented by its low sensitivity. The situation on the EDB was somewhat better for Asian/Pacific Islander beneficiaries. Here, sensitivity was 54.7 percent, correctly identifying only slightly more than half of this group. Specificity and NPV were both very high at 99.8 and 99.2, respectively. Even the PPV was respectable at 84.5 percent, and the Kappa coefficient at 0.66 was only slightly lower than for White beneficiaries, likely reflecting the lower sensitivity.

2.2   Development of the Algorithm

In light of the low sensitivity of the Hispanic and Asian/Pacific Islander race/ethnicity categories on the EDB, we employed a multi-stage process through which separate Hispanic and Asian/Pacific Islander imputation algorithms were developed. These algorithms used several pieces of information on the EDB including:

A. A variable that identified the language a beneficiary preferred CMS use when sending the Medicare Handbook. English, Spanish, and blank (no preference specified) were the only allowed values. This variable is referred to as LANGPREF.

B. A variable that identified the language a beneficiary requested the Social Security Administration (SSA) use when sending beneficiary notices. This variable was used by CMS for Medicare premium bills. English (for Puerto Rican zip codes only), Spanish, and blank (English assumed for non-Puerto Rican zip codes and Spanish assumed for Puerto Rican zip codes) were the only allowed values that HCFA supports. This code is referred to as LANGCD.

C. A variable that identified the source of a beneficiary's race/ethnicity code on the EDB (EDBRACE). This variable is referred to as RACESRC. Three values are allowed:

> A = Response from a one-time survey that was mailed to certain beneficiaries in 1997
>
> B = Indian Health Service
>
> Blank = Social Security Administration—Master Beneficiary Record (SSA-MBR) or SS-5 (NUMIDENT) or Railroad Retirement Board (RRB)

D. A variable that identified the state in which a beneficiary resides. We identified beneficiaries living in Hawaii and Puerto Rico.

The algorithms also used Hispanic (Word and Perkins, 1996) and Asian/Pacific Islander (Falkenstein and Word, 2002) surname lists developed by the U.S. Census Bureau. In the Hispanic surname list, Word and Perkins assign a percentage to each name representing the proportion of times a household headed by an individual with a particular Hispanic surname was indeed in an Hispanic household as reported to the Census. Falkenstein and Word had similar percentages for the Asian/Pacific Islander surname list.

We incorporated these pieces of information into a SAS program that, through an iterative process which differed slightly for Hispanics and Asians/Pacific Islanders, created an improved race/ethnicity variable (NEWRACE). The logic of the algorithms is described below.

A beneficiary was considered Hispanic (or Asian):

1. If the surname algorithm identified the beneficiary as Hispanic (Asian) at the stated inclusion level of 70 percent,

2. Otherwise, if the EDB coded the beneficiary as Hispanic (Asian),

3. Otherwise, if the person was a resident of Puerto Rico (Hawaii),

4. Otherwise, if the variable LANGCD indicated Spanish

5. Otherwise, if the beneficiary's first name had Hispanic (Asian) origins, and the surname, at the 50 percent inclusion level, identified the beneficiary as Hispanic (Asian)

A beneficiary was considered not Hispanic (Asian):

1. If not identified in the above steps,

2. Otherwise, if the variable LANGPREF indicated English,

3. Otherwise, if the variable RACESRC indicated the EDB's race code came from the 1995 survey and the EDB's race code is not "Hispanic," ("Asian")

4. Otherwise, if the variable RACESRC indicated the beneficiary's EDB race code came from the Indian Health Service.

2.3   Assessment of the Algorithm

Using the self-reported race/ethnicity data from the 2000-2002 Medicare CAHPS survey respondents as the gold standard, we assessed the results of applying the algorithms to the CAHPS respondents (i.e. the NEWRACE variable). We found the algorithms significantly improved the race/ethnicity categorization of Hispanic and Asian/Pacific Islander Medicare beneficiaries. As can be seen from Table 2.2, among Hispanic beneficiaries, sensitivity was 76.6 percent (improved from 29.5 percent), the Kappa coefficient was 0.79 (an increase from 0.43), and the other measures (specificity and predictive values) remained virtually unchanged. The improvement for Asian/Pacific Islander beneficiaries was equally impressive – sensitivity rose to 79.2 percent (from 54.7 percent), Kappa increased to 0.80 (from 0.66), and the other measures were not materially changed. Analysis of the improvements indicated that among both groups there were somewhat more males correctly identified than females (possibly due to intermarriage and surname changes for ethnic females), and more 65-74 year olds than those older than 74 (probably because there are more beneficiaries in the younger age group).

Table 2.2
Accuracy and agreement between NEWRACE and SELFRACE

NEWRACE	Accuracy and agreement measures for NEWRACE				
	Sensitivity	Specificity	Positive predictive value	Negative predictive value	Kappa
Asian/Pacific Islander	79.2	99.7	81.5	99.6	0.80
Hispanic	76.6	99.2	84.5	98.7	0.79

Source: NEWRACE is from the algorithms developed by RTI, and SELFRACE is from the Medicare CAHPS fee-for-service, managed care enrollee, and disenrollee surveys for 2000-2002. Table taken from the final report for CMS Contract Number 500-00-0024, Task 8 and has reformatted for this report from the project final report, *Health Disparities: Measuring Health Care Use and Access for Racial/Ethnic Populations* dated April 2005.

After demonstrating the clear advantage of using the Hispanic and Asian/Pacific Islander algorithms to improve the race/ethnicity categorization, the algorithms were combined and applied to all of the active records in the mid-2003 unloaded EDB.

2.4   Using the Algorithm to Provide an Improved Race/Ethnicity Variable

Upon combining the Hispanic and Asian/Pacific Islander naming algorithms and verifying the combined algorithm's success on the CAHPS data, we created the NEWRACE variable for the entire Medicare population found in the EDB. The first step was to obtain from CMS all 41.7 million records of active beneficiaries in the 10 segments of the unloaded EDB from mid-2003. After we had uploaded the EDB records, we were able to run the algorithm on the EDB records creating NEWRACE for each living beneficiary in the EDB.

Table 2.3 demonstrates the differences in the EDBRACE and NEWRACE variables for the entire population of active beneficiaries listed in the EDB. The number and percentage of Hispanic and A/PI beneficiaries increased, while they decreased for the White and Other race/ethnicity categories. The number and percent of Black beneficiaries also decreased slightly.

Table 2.3
Comparison of the distribution of race/ethnicity according to EDBRACE and NEWRACE for the entire EDB

	Original EDB race variable (EDBRACE)		New EDB race variable (NEWRACE)	
	Frequency	Percent	Frequency	Percent
White	35,141,623	84.2	33,424,922	80.1
Black	4,014,799	9.6	3,933,634	9.4
Hispanic	913,069	2.2	2,912,244	7.0
Asian/Pacific Islander (A/PI)	593,456	1.4	854,182	2.0
American Indian/Alaska Native (AI/AN)	137,989	0.3	136,498	0.3
Other	838,744	2.0	394,375	0.9
Unknown	101,095	0.2	85,254	0.2
Missing	1,631	0.0	1,297	0.0
Total	41,742,406	100.0	41,742,406	100.0

Source: EDBRACE is from Medicare EDB from mid-2003; and NEWRACE is the result of having run the combined surname algorithm on race/ethnicity in the Medicare EDB from mid-2003.

Table 2.4 shows that overall, 1,998,909[7] beneficiaries listed in the EDB had their race/ethnicity recoded to Hispanic as a result of using the combined improved naming algorithm. Most of these beneficiaries were originally classified in the EDB as White (83.5 percent), followed by Other/Unknown (11.1 percent), and Black (3.8 percent). Very few beneficiaries were originally coded as Asian/Pacific Islander (1.5 percent) or American Indian/Alaska Native (less than 0.05 percent). Overall, more female beneficiaries (1,068,033) than males (930,875) were recoded to Hispanic. This pattern holds true for White, Black, and Asian/Pacific Islander beneficiaries. The largest number of "new" Hispanic beneficiaries was created in the 65-to-74-year-old age group. This is true regardless of the beneficiaries' original EDB race/ethnicity code and gender. Not surprisingly, the 85-year- old-and-older age group had the fewest beneficiaries with their race/ethnicity recoded. This undoubtedly reflects the overall age distribution of Medicare beneficiaries.

---

[7] This excludes 266 beneficiaries who were originally coded as missing in the EDB but are now coded as Hispanics. Beneficiaries who were already coded as Hispanic in the EDB are also not included in this total.

Table 2.4

Distribution of "new" Hispanic beneficiaries (NEWRACE) according to their EDBRACE, gender, and age group

EDBRACE Gender and age group	White Number	Percent	Black Number	Percent	Asian/Pacific Islander Number	Percent	American Indian/ Alaska Native Number	Percent	Other or unknown Number	Percent	Total Number	Percent
Total	1,669,047	83.5	76,837	3.8	30,090	1.5	995	0.0	221,940	11.1	1,998,909	100.0
Male	767,952	82.5	36,070	3.9	12,499	1.3	520	0.1	113,834	12.2	930,875	100.0
Under 65	170,155	77.9	10,650	4.9	1,789	0.8	287	0.1	35,501	16.3	218,382	100.0
65-74	406,797	84.0	17,447	3.6	5,978	1.2	132	0.0	53,924	11.1	484,278	100.0
75-84	142,310	84.7	5,467	3.3	3,873	2.3	92	0.1	16,303	9.7	168,045	100.0
85 and Older	48,690	80.9	2,506	4.2	859	1.4	9	0.0	8,106	13.5	60,170	100.0
Female	901,095	84.4	40,767	3.8	17,591	1.6	475	0.0	108,105	10.1	1,068,033	100.0
Under 65	144,235	80.4	8,947	5.0	1,539	0.9	223	0.1	24,461	13.6	179,405	100.0
65-74	468,252	85.7	19,395	3.5	9,122	1.7	151	0.0	49,458	9.1	546,378	100.0
75-84	193,255	85.4	7,540	3.3	5,651	2.5	83	0.0	19,835	8.8	226,364	100.0
85 and Older	95,353	82.3	4,885	4.2	1,276	1.1	18	0.0	14,351	12.4	115,883	100.0

Source: EDBRACE is from Medicare EDB from mid-2003; and NEWRACE is the result of having run the combined surname algorithm on race/ethnicity in the Medicare EDB from mid-2003.

As can be seen from Table 2.5, among Asian/Pacific Islander beneficiaries, 290,748[8] were recoded as a result of using the combined improved naming algorithm. Unlike the Hispanic beneficiaries whose race/ethnicity was most often originally coded in the EDB as White, the majority of the new Asian/Pacific Islander beneficiaries were originally coded as Other/Unknown in the EDB. Exactly 82.0 percent of the newly coded Asian/Pacific Islander beneficiaries were originally coded as Other/Unknown. In addition, 16.4 percent were originally coded in the EDB as White, 1.5 percent as Black, and 0.2 percent as American Indian/Alaska Native. Note that we did not recode any beneficiaries to Asian/Pacific Islander who were originally coded as Hispanic in the EDB.

Table 2.5
Distribution of "new" Asian/Pacific Islander beneficiaries (NEWRACE) according to their EDBRACE, gender, and age group

EDBRACE Gender and age group	White		Black		American Indian/ Alaska Native		Other or Unknown		Total	
	Number	%	Number	%	Number	%	Number	%	Number	%
Total	47,654	16.4	4,328	1.5	496	0.2	238,270	82.0	290,748	100.0
Male	15,594	11.6	1,519	1.1	230	0.2	117,661	87.2	135,004	100.0
Under 65	2,392	11.6	473	1.1	49	0.2	9,809	87.2	12,723	100.0
65-74	7,858	9.0	770	0.9	114	0.1	78,366	90.0	87,108	100.0
75-84	4,157	15.6	226	0.8	60	0.2	22,241	83.3	26,684	100.0
85 and older	1,187	14.0	50	0.6	7	0.1	7,245	85.3	8,489	100.0
Female	32,060	20.6	2,809	1.8	266	0.2	120,609	77.4	155,744	100.0
Under 65	4,263	36.0	596	5.0	40	0.3	6,947	58.6	11,846	100.0
65-74	16,607	18.2	1,529	1.7	142	0.2	72,726	79.9	91,004	100.0
75-84	8,274	22.3	503	1.4	71	0.2	28,267	76.2	37,115	100.0
85 and older	2,916	18.5	181	1.1	13	0.1	12,669	80.3	15,779	100.0

Source: EDBRACE is from Medicare EDB from mid-2003; and NEWRACE is the result of having run the combined surname algorithm on race/ethnicity in the Medicare EDB from mid-2003.

With respect to gender and age, the Asian/Pacific Islander recodes were very similar to the Hispanic recodes. Across original EDB race/ethnicity and age groups, with the exception of the Asian/Pacific Islander group under 65 years of age, more females have been recoded to Asian/Pacific Islander than males. Overall 155,744 females were recoded compared to 135,004 males. As with Hispanic beneficiaries, the group of Asian/Pacific Islander beneficiaries 65 to 74 years of age was recoded most, while the group 85 and older was recoded least.

---

[8] This excludes 68 beneficiaries who were originally coded as missing in the EDB but are now coded as A/PI. Beneficiaries who were already coded as A/PI in the EDB are also not included in this total.

Overall, the combined improved naming algorithm recoded the race/ethnicity of 2,290,027 Medicare beneficiaries. Females and those 65 to 74 years of age were most often recoded to a new race/ethnicity when we used the combined improved naming algorithm on the full 10 segments of the unloaded EDB. For the new Hispanic beneficiaries, more were originally coded as White, compared to new Asian/Pacific Islander beneficiaries who were most often originally coded as Other/Unknown.

2.5   Geocoding Beneficiary Addresses to Link SES Data from the Census to the Beneficiaries in the EDB

Geocoding refers to the process of assigning a code number to each Medicare beneficiary's address that allows it to be linked to the U.S. Census data that describes characteristics of the beneficiary's place of residence. The primary reason to geocode the address of Medicare beneficiaries in the EDB is to enable the association of geographic-based U.S. Census measures of socioeconomic status (SES) with the beneficiaries, as there are now none on the EDB. While U.S. Census SES measures are not individual-level measures, they can be aggregated to specified geographic units, such as the census block, block group, tract, county, or state, that are associated with every beneficiary. We wanted to geocode beneficiary addresses so we could use the socioeconomic characteristics of their neighborhood (block group) to impute their SES. Examples of the SES characteristics from the Census that we chose to associate with Medicare beneficiaries were the median household income, the percentage of the population unemployed, the median value of owner occupied homes, and the percentage of the population below the federally-defined poverty level. Such characteristics can be used individually to examine the effects of SES or be combined in some way to more fully represent the concept of SES. As was discussed earlier, one of the objectives of this project was to create a multi-component measure of SES. The details of Census geography and related data elements are described more fully in the U.S. Census Bureau's Geographic Area Reference Manual located on-line at http://www.census.gov/geo/www/garm.html .

2.5.1   Address Cleaning

In order to link the beneficiaries in the EDB to the Census information available for the beneficiaries' residential area, there must be something in common on both records. The U.S. Census data is identified by a federal information processing standard (FIPS) code that can identify values for areas as small as blocks and block groups for the SES data in which we were interested. The beneficiary's residential area on the other hand is identified by an address. We needed some mechanism for efficiently translating the addresses in the EDB to FIPS codes that corresponded to those in the Census. We obtained a computer database product from GeoLytics Incorporated of East Brunswick, New Jersey – GeoCode program 2003 Version 1.02 – that was promoted by the manufacturer as being able to correctly assign FIPS codes to the level of Census blocks to addresses that were read into it.

Address information on Medicare beneficiaries is stored in the EDB in six address fields, each with a length of 22 characters. These address fields are generic, and labeled ADDRESS1, ADDRESS2, etc., and thus there is the potential for great variation in the type and order of information contained within the address fields. Upon examination, it appeared that the six fields were simply filled from left to right with whatever information had been collected about the beneficiary's address. The one exception was the beneficiary's zip code, which was always stored in the RESZIP field. However, the GeoLytics GeoCode program product requires that the beneficiaries' address input files be formatted in the following way:

STREET, CITY, STATE ZIP

The GeoCode program requires that STREET contains the street number and street name, separated by a space, with street name followed by a comma; then city followed by a comma, and then the two-letter state postal abbreviation code, a space, and the five digit zip code. It was a challenge and extremely time-consuming to extract, validate, and format these four pieces of information from the EDB address fields so they could be used as input for the GeoCode program. To meet this challenge, we developed the following procedures to apply to the EDB records:

1. Identify, for each beneficiary, what information is contained in each EDB address field

2. Extract the necessary information from the address fields, and create separate street, city, state, and zip code variables.

3. Verify that street, city, and state variables contain the information they are supposed to, check that the information is in the correct format, and, if not, put it in the correct format.

4. Output a text file (an ASCII text file, *.txt) in the proper format required as input for the GeoCode program.

5. Run the GeoCode program

   a. Input the address text file

   b. Output

      i. a text file summarizing the results of the address matching program

      ii. a database file (*.dbf) containing block IDs, error and accuracy codes, and other information related to the matched addresses.

6. Import the database file (*.dbf) into SAS, which transforms the *.dbf file to a *.sas7bdat file.

7. Merge the full transformed address file back onto the EDB records. This step adds a US Census-based geographic identifier (a string of FIPS codes) to each person-level beneficiary record.

This process was used to geocode the 10 separate segments of the unloaded EDB. The final step in the process allows the EDB to be linked to Census data files using the block group FIPS code that is common to both.

Time and resources did not permit us to identify and perform all of the necessary address preparation and verification activities manually on all 41 million-plus beneficiaries in the EDB. Instead, we used a random sample of addresses to identify incorrect patterns present in the beneficiaries' addresses in the EDB. Thus, we took a smaller batch of EDB records, specifically those EDB records corresponding to the 830,728 beneficiaries who responded to the CAHPS surveys we used earlier to develop the algorithm to improve on the EDB race/ethnicity coding to identify the various patterns exhibited in the EDB address fields. We developed SAS programs to extract, reformat, and validate the address information we needed, and then tested the performance of the GeoCode CD program. The following are the steps we performed to get the addresses from the EDB in good enough shape to run through the GeoCode program.

Identify and extract the information in each address field. EDB address fields could potentially follow many different patterns, and some did contain a good deal of superfluous or invalid information. Fortunately, the majority of records did follow a standard pattern:

1. ADDRESS1 contained the beneficiary's street address – both the street number and the street name. In some cases, this field also contained a direction (e.g., "East 1st Street," or "E 1st Street," or "1st Street E"), and/or an apartment number. [9]

2. ADDRESS2 contained either the beneficiary's city and state of residence or the beneficiary's apartment number

3. ADDRESS3, in cases where the ADDRESS2 field contained the apartment number or the like, contained the beneficiary's city and state of residence.

4. The last field with non-missing data typically contained the city and state of residence. So, in most cases, address fields 4, 5, and 6 were blank; a lesser number of cases had a blank for address field 3 as well.

The SAS program we wrote set the variable STREET equal to the EDB address field that should contain the street address (typically ADDRESS1). It also extracted separate CITY and STATE variables from the EDB address field that contained the city and state.

The RESZIP field in the EDB data contains the 9-digit Zip code. The SAS program dropped the last four digits of the EDB RESZIP variable, and created a new variable with the 5-digit Zip code (ZIP).

Verify the values and formats of STREET, CITY, and STATE. The first part of this step was completed prior to running addresses through the GeoCode program search engine. To verify that STREET and STATE contain the correct data, the SAS program checked for two things:

1. That the string of characters contained in the new variable, STREET, actually started with a number. This does not provide 100 percent verification, as it is possible for the string of characters contained in the variable STREET to start with a number, but not be an actual street address. However, this step does help ensure that STREET contains a street address.

2. That the string we identified as the state of residence (the new variable, STATE) was a valid two letter state postal abbreviation.

At this point, the STATE and ZIP variables were considered finalized. The remainder of the SAS algorithm focused on cleaning the STREET variable and ensuring that it was in the

---

[9] There are also several analogues to apartment number that appear in address fields, including suite number, lot number (in the case of mobile home parks), unit number, etc.

proper format. Before cleaning STREET, we dropped any cases where the GeoCode program would be unable to make a match, and for which we could obtain a match simply by reformatting the data. Dropped were addresses where:

1. The street address was missing

2. The beneficiary's state was invalid (as indicated by an invalid two letter state postal abbreviation which was often a foreign country), or they lived in Puerto Rico[10]

3. If the beneficiary's address was a rural route, an RFD, a P.O. Box, or Box number

For the remaining cases, CITY appeared to be relatively clean, and we did not attempt to reformat or validate that particular variable subsequent to dropping the cases listed above. Approximately 12.5 percent of the EDB records were dropped by this point, leaving us with about 87.5 percent of the records to which we applied further cleaning algorithms.

At this point, we began an iterative process of running small samples of the Medicare CAHPS survey addresses through the GeoCode address-matching process, identifying format-related problems in the street address field, and developing SAS code to repair the problems. Based on this testing process, we developed a series of six[11] "fixes," all of which were targeted to reformat specific anomalies that occurred regularly in the street address field. These fixes made repairs related to three basic elements of a street address that caused the address matching program to fail to find a valid match for what is a valid address:

1. Street address fields sometimes contained apartment, suite, lot, or unit numbers. While these are valid for mailing, the GeoCode program will return an error (i.e., "street not found") on an address containing one of these numbers. The first "fix" applied to the EDB address removed the apartment number (or analogue) out of the STREET field. This fix cleared the path for the subsequent five fixes that were applied to the STREET field.

2. In cases where the street NAME was actually a number (e.g., 25th Street, 1st Avenue, etc.), the Geocode program failed to find a valid match for the street if the suffix was missing from the numbered street. The suffix was almost always missing in the EDB address fields. We tested the suffix problem manually, and found that the simple addition of a suffix could, in many cases, turn a null match into an exact match. Numerical street names appear in a variety of patterns in the STREET variable, and four out of the five remaining fixes were designed to detect these patterns, and make the appropriate changes.

3. In some records, the street address contained what appeared to be a double street number – one 2- or 3-digit number, followed by a space, then another 2- or 3-digit number. We discovered that in some places, particularly Queens, NY, the space needs to be

---

[10] The GeoCode program does not match addresses in Puerto Rico.

[11] The "fixes" were numbered according to the order in which they were developed. However, the order in which they were applied in the SAS programs does not follow this numbering. Some fixes developed later (Fix 5, for example) had to be applied before earlier fixes.

replaced by a dash. In other places, however, it is unclear if the double number with a space is valid, or if the space should be deleted. In those cases, the double number was left as is.

For each fix, the SAS program outputs a text file listing, for each "fixed" record, the Medicare beneficiary's HIC number, the observation number, the address in it's original, "pre-fixed" format, the pattern of the new format, and the actual "fixed" address. This allowed us to check that the fix actually did what we expected it to, and it provides a record of the difference between the old addresses and the new addresses.

Output corrected addresses. The SAS program uses the PUT statement in conjunction with the FILE statement to output a single ASCII text file (*.txt) of addresses in the STREET, CITY, STATE ZIP format. This file contains all of the addresses that have been cleaned (100 percent of the records that were run through the fixes, or about 87.5 percent of the total number of beneficiary records). During testing we started with a CAHPS-matched EDB file with 830,728 records, which was reduced to 760,961 after the SAS program was run.

2.5.2 Running the GeoCode program

In testing the GeoCode program, we discovered that the program had a tendency for erratic performance. The help staff at GeoLytics seemed unable to explain the variations in performance. The primary problem was due to a lookup error—"failure to open data member" (eFOM). Between two and six percent of addresses we tested returned this error. Upon examination, we could not find any syntax errors that prevented these records from being successfully coded, and the technical support people at GeoLytics could not explain why these errors were occurring. However, we found that when we ran the addresses receiving the eFOM error code back through the GeoCode CD program a second time by themselves, they were matched at a 100 percent success rate.

The GeoLytics GeoCode CD program product allows the user to choose a variety of options that alter the balance between completeness of address coverage and speed of processing. In order to obtain maximum coverage, and thereby match the most addresses possible, we ran the GeoCode CD program with the following options turned on:

1. Allow phonetic match of state name

   – The geocoder phonetically matches the full state name in an address (but not an abbreviation).

2. Allow place-based ZIP code match

   – If a street is not found in a ZIP, the geocoder scans other ZIP codes associated with the place (typically a city or a town) for a match.

3. Allow phonetic match of street name

   – The geocoder uses a phonetic match for street names (e.g., an input address with the street name "Maine St." is considered a match with Main St. in the database).

4. Disregard parity for address match

- Normally, the geocoder matches even/odd addresses with even/odd address ranges. This option disregards this practice.

5. Allow closest address match

- The geocoder finds the closest address range to match the house number (rather than an exact one)

6. Allow fuzzy street type match

- The geocoder will match addresses with the same street name, even if the street types are different (e.g., Greenwood Drive is considered a match with Greenwood Road)

7. Geocode no matter what

- If it cannot find an exact match, the geocoder will assign to the address the census coordinates associated with the center of a ZIP code (ZIP centroid[12]), or the center of a state (state centroid).

The GeoCode program outputs two files as it runs – a text file (*.txt) summarizing the geocoder performance, the accuracy codes, and the error codes; and a database file (*.dbf) containing the fields selected by the user. For each database file, we selected the following fields[13]:

SEQNO	Sequential Number
ADDRESS	Input Address
ACCURACY	Accuracy and Error Codes
BLOCK	Matched Block Code
PLACE	Place FIPS Code
MCD	MCD (Minor Civil Division) Code
STATE	State FIPS Code
ZIP	ZIP Code for 2003
PLACENAME	Matched Place Name
AreaKey	Block Group Code

The sequential number field contains a number between 1 and n, where n is the total number of records processed by the program. The input address is the address in the STREET, CITY, STATE ZIP format constructed and output by the address cleaning SAS program. Accuracy and error codes are explained below. The matched block code is a string of fifteen

---

[12] The centroid of a 5-digit ZIP code area is the balance point of the polygon formed by its boundaries. The centroid is calculated based on the coordinate extremes of the polygon.

[13] One field we did not include, the MATCH field, contained the full address that the GeoCode search engine determined to be the closest match to the input address. We had intended to include this field, but during the testing phase, we discovered problems with the MATCH field that led to major problems when trying to transform the *.dbf files into SAS files.

digits that indicates, respectively, an individual's state (2 digit FIPS code), county (3 digit FIPS code), census tract (6 digit FIPS code), and block (4 digit FIPS code, the first digit in the 4-digit string indicates the block group). The full string constitutes a unique, block-level identifier. Any persons living within the same block will have the same matched block code. Place indicates the city or town FIPS code, and MCD indicates the Minor Civil Division code. The area key is basically a substring of the matched block code that contains the first twelve, rather than the full fifteen digits, and constitutes a unique block group-level identifier.

2.5.3 Summary of GeoCode program accuracy codes

Failure details. The geocoding process can fail for a number of reasons, including setup or programmatic errors, a missing database entry, or an invalid input address. Failures fall under two general categories: syntax/lookup errors and programmatic/setup errors. Failed GeoCode results are indicated by error codes, which are summarized in Tables 2.6 and 2.7.

Table 2.6
GeoCode program syntax and lookup errors

Error Code	Error Message
eIHN	Missing or invalid house number*
eISt	Missing or invalid street name*
eITy	Missing or invalid street type
eINa	Missing or invalid city name
eISN	Missing or invalid state name/abbrev*
eIZI	Missing or invalid ZIP code*
eIAd	Incomplete or malformed address*
eUAF	Unknown address format
eMiA	Missing address
eNZI	Failed to lookup ZIP code
eANF	Address not found
eSNF	Street not found

*Errors encountered while geocoding EDB addresses.

Source: GeoLytics Incorporated of East Brunswick, New Jersey – GeoCode CD program 2003, Version 1.02.

Table 2.7
GeoCode program programmatic and setup errors

Error Code	Error Message
eGNO	GeoCode has not been opened
eFOD	Failed to open database
eFOF	Failed to open data file NAME
eFOM	Failed to open data member NAME*
eMiF	Missing file NAME
eGOF	General open failure, file NAME
eFA1	Failed to allocate memory
eNAS	No address data for state NAME*
eNSZ	No data for state-zip NAME
eSSO	String size overflow
eOKI	Output file kind invalid NAME
eOF1	Output failure NAME
eOLI	Output field list invalid NAME

*Errors encountered while geocoding EDB addresses.

Source: GeoLytics Incorporated of East Brunswick, New Jersey – GeoCode CD program 2003, Version 1.02.

Success details. The GeoCode program also indicates how successful it has been in matching addresses to FIPS codes. In addition to indicating accurate or exact matches, it indicates what kinds of "adjustments" it made to successfully match the address to a place with a FIPS code. Successful match details are presented in Table 2.8. Some successful results will generate accuracy codes indicating that the geocoder could only code the address by using some of the fallback matching options described above. Its worth noting that GeoCode CD may employ more than one of these fallback matching options to find a match for a particular address.

Table 2.8
GeoCode program accuracy codes and messages

Accuracy Code	Accuracy Message
aNP1	Place not found*
aNPa	Address match with no parity*
aCAd	Closest address match*
aFTy	Fuzzy street type match*
aPhM	Phonetic match*
aNMa	No match found
aNMP	No match performed
aPBZ	Place-based ZIP match*
aSpC	Spelling corrected*
aStC	State centroid used*
aSEn	Street end used*
aZIC	ZIP centroid used*
aInD	Inaccurate direction*

*Accuracy options encountered while geocoding EDB addresses.

Source: GeoLytics Incorporated of East Brunswick, New Jersey – GeoCode CD program 2003, Version 1.02

Test results using the GeoCode program on the CAHPS sample addresses. Table 2.9 below summarizes the error and accuracy results from the CAHPS sample test file. It indicates that 8.4 percent of the 830,728 CAHPS sample addresses taken from the EDB were dropped because they were uncodeable by the GeoCode program for some reason, very often for having a box number instead of a street address. It also shows that of the remaining 760,961 addresses (91.6 percent of the original total), all but four-tenths of a percent (0.4 percent) were successfully geocoded. The process we followed in this test yielded an overall total successful match of 91.2 percent of the EDB addresses to Census block group level FIPS codes.

Table 2.9
Summary of GeoCode error and accuracy results for the CAHPS test file

	CAHPS/EDB Test File	
	Number	Percent
Original number of records	830,728	100.0
Number of records dropped (uncodeable)	69,767	8.4
Addresses processed	760,961	91.6
...Successfully geocoded (first iteration)	719,220	94.5
...Successfully geocoded eFOM records (second iteration)	38,322	5.0
...Total failed	3,419	0.4
GeoCode success rate	757,542	99.6
Percent total test file records matched		91.2
Success details*		
Accurate Match	477,746	62.8
Place Not Found	77,273	10.2
Address match with no parity	5,931	0.8
Closest address match	37,984	5.0
Fuzzy street type match	86,701	11.4
Phonetic match	37,847	5.0
Place-based ZIP match	16,519	2.2
Spelling corrected	0	0.0
State centroid used	905	0.1
Street end used	3,871	0.5
ZIP centroid used	63,031	8.3
Inaccurate direction	20,525	2.7
Failure details		
Failed due to syntax error	3,418	0.4
...Missing or invalid house number	3,367	0.4
...Missing or invalid state name/abbreviation	0	0.0
...Missing or invalid ZIP code	47	0.0
...Incomplete or malformed address	4	0.0
Failed due to lookup error	38,323	5.0
...Failed to open data member (eFOM)	38,322	5.0
...No address data for state	1	0.0

*Note: Success detail categories reflect distribution of accuracy codes. These codes are NOT mutually exclusive. Some addresses can have up to four accuracy codes associated with them.

Source: Result of running GeoCode CD program 2003 Version 1.02 on addresses from Medicare EDB from mid-2003 for respondents to the Medicare CAHPS fee-for-service, managed care enrollee, and disenrollee surveys for 2000-2002.

2.5.4 Application of the GeoCode Program Processing to the Full EDB

We obtained the 10 segments of the full unloaded EDB from CMS in mid-2003. Because each segment of the EDB contained more than four million beneficiary records, we processed each segment separately, first extracting the addresses and other necessary identification variables from the EDB, correcting the addresses using the SAS programs we developed, and finally running them through the GeoCode program. Each segment of the EDB was run through the GeoCode program separately. The program took from 16 to 36 hours to process and match the more than four million records contained in each segment. As indicated above in the description of the test results on the CAHPS sample addresses, it was necessary to rerun the addresses with an eFOM error that failed to match on the first iteration, and virtually all of them were successfully matched on the second iteration through the GeoCode program.

Run EDB segments through the GeoCode program. The results of the GeoCode program processing are summarized in Table 2.10 for all 10 segments of the unloaded EDB combined. The results were extremely similar for each of the 10 segments. Overall, 86.8 percent of the 41,742,407 addresses of Medicare beneficiaries were processed through the Geocode program. Ninety-nine and two tenths percent of the addresses that were processed (or 36,223,053) were successfully matched to a FIPS code that included the block group. As Table 2.8 shows, 61 percent of the matches made were exact with the addresses that were input.

Import Geocode output files and merge with EDB records. We used PROC IMPORT in SAS 8.2 to transform the database (*.dbf) files produced by the GeoCode program into SAS data files (*.sas7bdat). Using the ADDRESS field we prepared as input from the EDB to the GeoCode program as the common key (common to the EDB and the GeoCode output), we merged the output files (containing Census-based geographic identifiers including the AreaKey number string that identifies block groups) onto the EDB records.

2.5.5 Results of Geo-coding the Sample of 1.96 Million Medicare Beneficiaries

The sample of 1.96 million Medicare fee-for-service beneficiaries is a subset of the beneficiaries geocoded from the mid-2003 EDB. The results of the geocoding for the 1.96 million are presented in Table 2.11. While the table indicates that 81 percent (1,588,121 out of 1,960,121) of the addresses for the sample members were successfully geocoded, this was with allowing the use of ZIP code and state centroid when there was no other way to achieve a successful match of the input address to a Census-listed address. It should be noted that we did rerun unmatched addresses from the mid-2003 EDB as well as those that changed from the mid-2003 through the Geocode CD in the hope of more completely and correctly geocoding sample members.

We know from analyses performed in sub-task one of this task order that most of the state centroid matches (4,090) are not true matches at all, but forced to the state centroid by the GeoCode CD program on addresses that are foreign. The same may be true of some of the Zip (159,217) centroid matches as well. We feel very confident saying, however, that based upon our validation of address block group matching against the Census, that the true match rate at the block group level for the sample is most likely at least 75 percent.

Table 2.10
Summary of GeoCode error and accuracy codes for the 10 segments of the EDB combined

	Sums	Percent
Original number of records	41,742,407	100.0
Number of records excluded (uncodeable)	5,223,766	12.5
Addresses processed	36,518,641	87.5
...Successfully geocoded (First Iteration)	35,108,329	96.1
...Successfully geocoded eFOM records (second iteration)	1,114,724	3.1
...Total failed	295,588	0.8
Geocoding success rate	36,223,053	99.2
Percent total EDB records matched		86.8
Success details*		
Accurate match	20,028,633	61.0
Place not found	3,216,868	9.8
Address match with no parity	281,554	0.9
Closest address match	1,821,893	5.5
Fuzzy street type match	3,919,792	11.9
Phonetic match	1,752,858	5.3
Place-based ZIP match	799,836	2.4
Spelling corrected	10	0.0
State centroid used	47,252	0.1
Street end used	181,270	0.6
ZIP centroid used	2,972,274	9.0
Inaccurate direction	1,027,377	3.1
Failure details		
Failed due to syntax error	262,176	0.8
...Missing or invalid house number	175,561	0.5
...Missing or invalid state name/abbr	4	0.0
...Missing or invalid ZIP code	86,335	0.3
...Incomplete or malformed address	276	0.0
Failed due to lookup error	1,022,267	3.4
...Failed to open data member (eFOM)	1,018,483	3.4
...No address data for state	3,784	0.0

*Note: Success detail categories reflect distribution of accuracy codes. These codes are NOT mutually exclusive. Some addresses can have up to four accuracy codes associated with them.

Source: Result of running GeoCode CD program 2003, Version 1.02 on addresses from Medicare EDB from mid-2003.

Table 2.11
Success with Geocoding of the Medicare Beneficiaries Included in the RTI Sample of 1.96 Million

Total Sample	1,960,121
Successfully geocoded	1,588,607
GeoCoding Success Rate	**81.0%**
Success Details	
Exact Match	920,390
Other Accuracy Code	504,910
Zip Centroid	159,217
State Centroid	4,090

Source: Result for sample of 1.96 million of running GeoCode CD program 2003, Version 1.02 on addresses from Medicare EDB from mid-2003.

2.6   Selection of a Sample of 1.96 Million Medicare Beneficiaries from the EDB

We selected a nationally representative stratified, simple, random sample of traditional fee-for-service Medicare beneficiaries designed to over-sample minorities to create and validate an SES index (discussed in the next section of this report), prepare tabulations (discussed in the following section), and conduct multivariate analyses (discussed in the final section).This sample was initially drawn for analyses performed in the previous task order contract and reported on in the report titled *Health Disparities: Measuring Health Care Use and Access for Racial/Ethnic Populations* (2005).

We drew the sample from the full 10 segments of the mid-2003 unloaded EDB. To be eligible for inclusion in the sample, beneficiaries must have been enrolled in traditional fee-for-service (FFS) Medicare (Part A, Part B, or both) for the full 12 months of the 2002 calendar year and not have been enrolled in a Group Health Organization at all during the 2002 calendar year. In addition, beneficiaries must have been alive for the full 12 months of calendar year 2002. We set these criteria to allow the maximum opportunity (period of time) for beneficiaries to submit claims documenting their use of preventive and other Medicare covered services.

Table 2.12 presents a distribution of the beneficiaries included on the EDB eligible for the sample by their NEWRACE (their race/ethnicity code resulting from the use of the naming algorithm created by RTI) and by EDBRACE (their race/ethnicity code on the EDB before using the naming algorithm), respectively.

The primary sampling goal at the time this sample was selected was to have sufficient sample size to provide equally accurate and precise estimates of health care utilization for the different racial/ethnic groups. We therefore stratified by race/ethnicity and sampled such that, to the extent possible, the same number of Medicare beneficiaries would be included in the sample in each of the different racial/ethnic groups. This meant that the sample included disproportionately more minorities than their representation in Medicare. The sampling rates based on the NEWRACE code was 11 percent for Black Medicare beneficiaries, 1.2 percent for White, 26 percent for Hispanic, 71 percent for Asian/Pacific Islander, and 100 percent of American Indian/Alaska Native, Other, and Unknown.

Table 2.12
Distribution of Medicare fee-for-service beneficiaries believed eligible for the study sample by NEWRACE and EDBRACE

Race/Ethnicity Category	Frequency of NEWRACE	Frequency of EDBRACE
Non-Hispanic White	25,907,883	27,091,613
Non-Hispanic Black	3,025,397	3,087,034
Hispanic	2,081,123	730,147
Non-Hispanic Asian/Pacific Islander	592,010	453,950
Non-Hispanic American Indian/Alaska Native	121,024	122,156
Non-Hispanic Other	183,242	412,198
Unknown	61,567	75,148
Total	31,972,246	31,972,246

Source: EDBRACE is from the Medicare EDB from mid-2003 and NEWRACE is the result of running the algorithm on those same beneficiaries from the Medicare EDB from mid-2003.

These sampling rates produced the sample presented in Table 2.13 according to NEWRACE and EDBRACE .

Table 2.13
Distribution of Medicare fee-for-service beneficiaries selected for the study sample by NEWRACE and EDBRACE

Race/Ethnicity Category	Frequency of NEWRACE	Frequency of EDBRACE
Non-Hispanic White	333,334	658,279
Non-Hispanic Black	333,334	350,879
Hispanic	545,643	191,402
Non-Hispanic Asian/Pacific Islander	421,859	312,785
Non-Hispanic American Indian/Alaska Native	121,024	121,496
Non-Hispanic Other	183,242	299,015
Unknown	61,567	66,147
Total	2,000,003	2,000,003

Source: EDBRACE is from the Medicare EDB from mid-2003 and NEWRACE is the result of running the algorithm on those same beneficiaries from the Medicare EDB from mid-2003.

White and Black beneficiaries have the same size sample, while American Indian/Alaska Native, Other, and Unknown have fewer, and Hispanics and Asians/Pacific Islanders have slightly more. As already mentioned above, our sampling goals were to have as close to equal sample for each race/ethnicity as possible in order to provide equally accurate and precise estimates of utilization for each of the racial/ethnic groups. Thus, we sampled 100 percent of the American Indian/Alaska Native, Other, and Unknown beneficiaries and therefore could not get them any closer to the White and Black numbers. In the case of Hispanic and Asian/Pacific Islanders beneficiaries, however, we increased their allocation in the sample slightly because we wanted the estimates to be as close to equally precise across the race/ethnicity categories when the NEWRACE code was used rather than the EDBRACE. (The number of Asian/Pacific Islanders and Hispanics would have dropped whenever the EDBRACE code was used instead of the NEWRACE and so would the precision of the estimates; therefore, we decided to sample more Asian/Pacific Islanders and Hispanics to maintain the precision of the estimates).

After the sample was selected, we cross-referenced it with CMS's denominator file as a final check on eligibility and discovered that slightly less than two percent of the selected sample, spread proportionately across the racial/ethnic groups, did not meet all of our desired sample eligibility criteria – alive and enrolled in fee-for-service Medicare for the entire year. We identified and discarded the ineligibles from the sample and recalculated the weights of the remaining sample to correctly represent the intended population of eligible Medicare fee-for-service beneficiaries. Table 2.14 presents the final number of sampled beneficiaries by NEWRACE and EDBRACE.

Table 2.14
Distribution of final study sample of selected Medicare fee-for-service beneficiaries by NEWRACE and EDBRACE

Race/Ethnicity Category	Frequency of NEWRACE	Frequency of EDBRACE
Non-Hispanic White	329,954	647,653
Non-Hispanic Black	328,246	345,559
Hispanic	534,196	187,920
Non-Hispanic Asian/Pacific Islander	415,190	308,890
Non-Hispanic American Indian/Alaska Native	120,557	121,025
Non-Hispanic Other	171,032	283,603
Unknown	60,946	65,471
Total	1,960,121	1,960,121

Source: EDBRACE is from the Medicare EDB from mid-2003 and NEWRACE is the result of running the algorithm on those same beneficiaries from the Medicare EDB from mid-2003.

Table 2.15 contains the distribution of the weighted number of Medicare beneficiaries contained in the EDB who are represented in the sample distributed by the NEWRACE and EDBRACE variables.

Table 2.15
Distribution of weighted study sample of Medicare beneficiaries by
NEWRACE and EDBRACE

Race/Ethnicity Category	Frequency of NEWRACE	Frequency of EDBRACE
Non-Hispanic White	25,645,178	26,779,400
Non-Hispanic Black	2,979,217	3,053,618
Hispanic	2,037,463	720,664
Non-Hispanic Asian/Pacific Islander	582,651	449,914
Non-Hispanic American Indian/Alaska Native	120,557	121,818
Non-Hispanic Other	171,032	397,030
Unknown	60,946	74,600
Total	31,597,044	31,597,044

Source: EDBRACE is from the Medicare EDB from mid-2003 and NEWRACE is the result of running the algorithm on those same beneficiaries from the Medicare EDB from mid-2003.

2.7 Identifying the Top 10 Metropolitan Statistical Areas (MSAs) for Asian/Pacific Islander and Hispanic Elderly Population

In addition to the tabular investigations to be performed of racial and ethnic disparities in health care utilization by Medicare beneficiaries at the national level, this task was intended to provide additional insight into racial and ethnic disparities in smaller areas with high concentrations of elderly Asians and Hispanics. Rather than target states with large Asian and Hispanic residents, the task called for us to identify metropolitan statistical areas (MSAs) in which there would potentially be large numbers and high concentrations of Asian/Pacific Islander and Hispanic Medicare beneficiaries. The purpose for looking at utilization in selected MSAs was to investigate whether, in areas where members of these minorities were a significant segment of the health care market, there were fewer disparities in services used and greater similarities in health care use to that of non-Hispanic Whites. It is important to keep in mind that in such analyses, the number of Medicare beneficiaries in the sample and the frequency with which the services were used for the MSAs studied had to be adequately large to achieve statistically reliable estimates.

To investigate this issue, we identified the ten MSAs, or the Primary MSAs within Consolidated MSAs, from the 2000 US Census with the largest number of persons 65 years of age and older who identified themselves in the Census as Asian, Native Hawaiian, or Pacific Islanders. The MSAs we identified are listed in Table 2.16 for Asians/Native Hawaiians /Pacific Islanders. We did the same for persons who were identified as Hispanic or Latino. Those MSAs are identified and listed in Table 2.17 for Hispanics/Latinos. The MSAs are listed according to the number of elderly Asian/Native Hawaiians/Pacific Islander and Hispanic/Latino population in each.

When we prepared the tabulations for this report, it became apparent that the two sets of 10 MSAs reduced to a single set of 16, because four MSAs were common to both lists. The MSAs common to both lists are Los Angeles, New York, Chicago, and San Diego.

35

Table 2.16
Top 10 MSAs for Number of Asian/Native Hawaiian/Pacific Islander Population 65 Years of Age and Older: 2000

Metropolitan Statistical Area	Total population: Total	Total population: Asian/NH/PI	Percent of total population who are Asian/NH/PI	Total population: 65+	Asian/NH/PI population, 65+	Percent o 65+ pers who a Asian/NF
Los Angeles--Long Beach, CA PMSA	9,519,338	1,164,553	12.2%	926,673	120,811	13.0%
Honolulu, HI MSA	876,156	481,051	54.9%	117,737	85,429	72.6%
New York, NY PMSA	9,314,235	851,460	9.1%	1,109,821	62,887	5.7%
San Francisco, CA PMSA	1,731,183	406,087	23.5%	227,628	53,814	23.6%
Oakland, CA PMSA	2,392,557	411,819	17.2%	254,863	36,265	14.2%
San Jose, CA PMSA	1,682,585	435,868	25.9%	160,527	31,926	19.9%
Orange County, CA PMSA	2,846,289	395,723	13.9%	280,763	30,181	10.7%
Chicago, IL PMSA	8,272,768	384,932	4.7%	888,505	24,964	2.8%
San Diego, CA MSA	2,813,833	263,363	9.4%	313,750	22,593	7.2%
Washington, DC--MD--VA--WV PMSA	4,923,153	332,919	6.8%	446,288	20,703	4.6%
Total in 10 MSAs	44,372,097	5,127,775	11.6%	4,726,555	489,573	10.4%

Source: U.S. Census Bureau, Census 2000 Summary File 1 (SF 1) 100-Percent Data, Table P12. Available online at: http://factfinder.census.gov/servlet/DTGeoSearchByListServlet?ds_name=DEC_2000_SF1_U&_lang=en&_ts=16455392 5612

Table 2.17
Top 10 MSAs for Number of Hispanic/Latino Population 65 Years of Age and Older: 2000

Metropolitan Statistical Area	Total population: Total	Total population: Hispanic or Latino	Percent of total population who are Hispanic or Latino	Total population: 65+	Hispanic Population, 65+	Percent of all 65+ population who are Hispanic or Latino
Los Angeles--Long Beach, CA PMSA	9,519,338	4,242,213	44.6%	926,673	187,447	20.2%
Miami, FL PMSA	2,253,362	1,291,737	57.3%	300,552	184,625	61.4%
New York, NY PMSA	9,314,235	2,339,836	25.1%	1,109,821	146,219	13.2%
San Antonio, TX MSA	1,592,383	816,037	51.2%	169,748	59,486	35.0%
Riverside--San Bernardino, CA PMSA	3,254,821	1,228,962	37.8%	342,423	49,499	14.5%
Chicago, IL PMSA	8,272,768	1,416,584	17.1%	888,505	44,620	5.0%
El Paso, TX MSA	679,622	531,654	78.2%	66,073	43,210	65.4%
Houston, TX PMSA	4,177,646	1,248,586	29.9%	311,213	37,968	12.2%
San Diego, CA MSA	2,813,833	750,965	26.7%	313,750	34,149	10.9%
McAllen--Edinburg--Mission, TX MSA	569,463	503,100	88.3%	55,274	32,847	59.4%
Total	42,447,471	14,369,674	33.9%	4,484,032	820,070	18.3%

Source: U.S. Census Bureau, Census 2000 Summary File 1 (SF 1) 100-Percent Data, Table P12. Available online at: http://factfinder.census.gov/servlet/DTGeoSearchByListServlet?ds_name=DEC_2000_SF1_U&_lang=en&_ts=16455392 5612

3. CREATING AND VALIDATING AN INDEX OF SOCIOECONOMIC STATUS

3.1   Introduction

Over the years, there has been considerable empirical evidence accumulated that indicates in the US that health status, mortality, and health services use differ by what has been referred to variously as socioeconomic status, social class, social position or SES. (Braverman et al. 2005) More recently, there has been a growing unease about the accumulation of evidence on the extent of variation in health status, mortality, and health services use that is associated with race and ethnicity (Krieger et al., 2005). While they are different, it is unfortunate that socioeconomic status and race/ethnicity are not independent of one another in their association with health status, mortality, and health services use. This has at times led to the mistaken use of race/ethnicity as a surrogate measure of socioeconomic status.

Because of this, it is particularly important to try to separate the influences of socioeconomic status (SES) and race/ethnicity on health and utilization of health services in our empirical research. Only then will it be possible for policymakers to identify where to place their priorities in the development of ameliorative interventions – to overcome the socioeconomic barriers to accessing timely, appropriate, and good quality care, the sub-cultural values and restricted world view that keep some minorities from taking full advantage of the services available to them, or the prejudice against minorities of providers and the health care system. As we indicated earlier, the first objective of this project is to create and validate a measure of SES to include in analyses of racial/ethnic health care disparities in the use of covered services by Medicare beneficiaries.

Our interest in this issue arises from the use of Medicare claims in the study of racial/ethnic disparities. Medicare beneficiaries enrolled in the fee-for-service program present an ideal opportunity to study racial/ethnic disparities in health status, mortality, and health services use because they have similar health care coverage. The Medicare enrollment database (EDB) contains person-specific information on the demographic characteristics – age, gender, race/ethnicity – of beneficiaries. It also includes information on whether beneficiaries receive additional Government benefits – ranging from help paying their share of premiums to benefits not included in regular Medicare – due to their low income level. It does not, however, include any person-level measures that are typically considered indicators of socioeconomic status.

The EDB does contain residential address information for beneficiaries that, while not in a form that is immediately useable, can with some reasonable effort be transformed into a geocode that corresponds to US Census designated areas (e.g., block groups, tracts, municipalities, counties, ZIP code tabulation areas, states, divisions, regions). These areas have some well-accepted indicators of socioeconomic status reported at least every 10 years. In fact, a literature has developed in Epidemiology, Social Medicine, and Medical Sociology that has established the relevance of SES measures at the level of meaningful homogeneous social aggregates like neighborhoods and communities. It has been shown that such social aggregates reflect common culture, behavior, norms, and values in response to selected symptoms of ill health, health care seeking behavior, as well as demonstrating likely differences in access to services, quality of available care, and discrimination in the provision of services.

3.2   Prior Work As The Starting Point

We began our SES index development activity based on the work of Dr. Nancy Krieger and colleagues from the Harvard University School of Public Health working on the Public Health Disparities Geocoding Project (Krieger, et al, 2003a) She and her colleagues have published extensively on the development and use of socioeconomic measures to understand disparities in health and health care (Krieger, et al, 2003b; Krieger, et al, 2005; Krieger, et al, 2002a; Krieger et al., 2002b). They have noted the absence of person level socioeconomic status measures in many research areas relying on analyses of administrative data and have promoted the practice of geocoding addresses and the use of area-based measures of socioeconomic status.

Socioeconomic status is a multidimensional concept. Among the dimensions typically associated with SES are occupational status, educational achievement, income, poverty, and wealth. Krieger has identified and employed a number of Census measures that are available to measure many of the dimensions associated with socioeconomic status (SES). These include for occupational status: percentage of the population in the working class (based on percent of persons employed in non-supervisory positions in 8 of 13 occupational groups) and the percentage of the labor force that is unemployed; for the income dimension: the median household income, the percentage of households with income below half of the national median income, and the percentage with household incomes more than four times the national median income; for poverty: the percentage of the population below the Federal poverty level; for wealth: the percentage of households with owner occupied homes valued at four times or more of the national median home value; for the educational dimension: the percentage of the adult population with less than a 12th grade education, and the percentage with at least four years of college education; and crowding: percentage of households with one or more persons per room. Krieger has developed composite socioeconomic status measures based on principal components factor analyses of these and related Census variables for Zip code areas, census tracts, and census block groups in several states. In addition, she and her colleagues have used them in analyses of birth, death, and other public health statistics that can be associated with geographic areas (addresses and geocodes).

As we indicate earlier in this document, while it is possible to analyze Medicare claims to investigate the presence of racial and ethnic disparities in health care utilization, the lack of a readily available measure of socio-economic status to separate the impact of SES from race and ethnicity has been a real limitation to identifying health care disparities associated exclusively with race/ethnicity. It was to create such a measure to make this kind of analysis possible that this sub-task was conceived. The first objective of it was to establish whether it was possible to create a reasonably good single composite measure of SES that could be assigned to individual beneficiaries based on a number of measures of residential area characteristics available from the 2000 US Census. Because we did not have person-level measures of the previously mentioned SES dimension indicators, we instead geocoded each Medicare beneficiary's residential address and identified a FIPS code for that address that links to Census data available at the block group level.

Block groups are a cluster of census blocks having the same first digit of the four-digit identifying numbers within a common census tract. Block groups generally contain between 600 and 3,000 people, with an optimum size of 1,500 people. We have chosen to use block groups rather than the smaller block unit because it is the lowest level Census geographic unit for which we have available the kind of economic measures for the area whose characteristics we can use to represent Medicare beneficiaries' residential areas.

3.3   Development of the SES Index

The first step in the process of creating a composite SES index for Medicare beneficiaries was to perform a principal components type of factor analysis. We chose to use this type of analysis to quantify into a single index value the contributions of a set of several SES related measures thought to contribute to the measurement of the primary underlying dimension of the measures, which we will refer to as SES. It was our intention that the index we were attempting to produce would be based on the first principal component emerging from the analysis, because the first principal component would account for the greatest variation in the analyzed measures among the block groups and be independent of any other components that might emerge subsequent to it in the analysis.

We performed a principal component analysis on a set of seven measures identified and used previously by Krieger (Krieger, et al, 2003a). These measures are on their face considered related to, and are at times used as proxies for, SES. The measures we included in the principal components analysis were: (1) as a measure of occupation, the percentage of persons in the block group who are 16 years of age and older and in the labor force but are unemployed; (2) as a measure of income, the percentage of persons in the block group living below the federal poverty level; (3) as a related measure of income, a standardized[14] measure of the median household income in the block group; (4) as a measure of wealth, a standardized measure of the median value of owner-occupied dwellings in the Block Group; (5) as a measure of educational attainment, the percentage of persons 25 years of age or older with less than a 12th grade education; (6) as a second measure of educational attainment, the percentage of persons 25 years of age or older who completed at least four years of college; and (7) as a measure of crowding related to wealth (based on fact that lower income persons have on average more persons per room than wealthier persons who typically have larger homes), the percentage of households that average one or more persons per room.

We analyzed these variables across the entire set of 211,267 U.S. Census block groups that had all seven measures available. The results of the principal components analysis of the seven SES variables, using data from the block groups, are presented in Table 3.1. To determine whether the first principal component appropriate accounts for most of the variance common to the seven measures, we examined the eigenvalues. A common rule of thumb is that one principal component (in this case the first one is the only one in which we are interested) is adequate to represent the common aspect of the measures when the ratio of the first to second eigenvalue is at least three. In our analyses, this ratio was equal to 2.98, or rounded to 3.0, because the first eigenvalue was 3.85 and the second one was 1.29. Therefore, we were satisfied with extracting only the first principal component.

---

[14] The standardization was accomplished by subtracting the mean of the distribution from each value and dividing by the standard deviation of the distribution.

Table 3.1
Principal Components Analysis of Seven SES Measures: Based on Block-Group Data for 2000 US Census (N = 211,267)

Construct	Measure	Definition	Principal Components Loading
Occupation			
	Unemployment	Percentage of persons aged 16 years or older in the labor force who are unemployed (and actively seeking work)	-0.66
Income			
	Below US poverty line	Percentage of persons below the federally defined poverty line	-0.79
	Median income*	Median household income	0.85
Wealth			
	Property values*	Median value of owner-occupied homes	0.64
Education			
	Low education	Percentage of persons aged ≥ 25 years with less than a 12th-grade education	-0.84
	High education	Percentage of persons aged ≥ 25 years with at least 4 years of college	0.79
Housing			
	Crowded households	Percentage of households containing one or more person per room	-0.56

* These variables are standardized to have values ranging from 0 to 100.

Note: Values of loadings are multiplied by -1 so that higher values for the composite scores represent higher SES levels.

The loadings of each of the variables on the first principal component are also displayed in Table 3.1. The loadings can be interpreted as measures of association between the individual measures and the first principal component which we are calling socioeconomic status or SES. The associations are reasonably high and they all run in the anticipated directions. The positive signs indicate that the following block group measures are associated with higher SES: larger percentages of more highly educated, higher median home values, and higher median household incomes. The block group measures with negative signs indicate that those are associated with lower SES: higher percentages of unemployed persons, larger percentages of persons below the federal poverty level, greater percentages of persons with less than a 12th grade education, and higher percentages of households with one or more persons per room.

We attempted to compute SES index scores for all 211,267 block groups in the U.S. according to the formula in Figure 3.1, but there were 3,462 for which the data were missing for some measures and an SES index could not be calculated. The SES index scores were derived by multiplying the measure's values times the respective weights estimated by the principal components analysis and summing them.

Figure 3.1
Scoring Algorithm for SES Index

SES Index Score = $50 + (-0.07*crowded) + (0.08*prop100) + (-0.10*pct\_poverty) +$

$(0.11*hhinc100) + (0.10*high\_educ) + (-0.11*low\_educ) +$

$(-0.08*pct\_unemp)$

Abbreviations:

- crowded = Percentage of households containing one or more person per room
- prop100 = Median value of owner-occupied values, standardized to range from 0-100
- pct_poverty = Percentage of persons below the federally defined poverty line
- hhinc100 = Median household income, standardized to range from 0-100
- high_educ = Percentage of persons aged ≥ 25 years with at least 4 years of college
- low_educ = Percentage of persons aged ≥ 25 years with less than a 12th-grade education
- pct_unemp = Percentage of persons aged 16 years or older in the labor force who are unemployed (and actively seeking work)

The distribution of the SES scores for the block groups is presented in Table 3.2. While the SES scores were calculated to theoretically range from 0 to 100, they actually only ranged from 21 to 78. The scores were grouped as closely as possible into quartiles. The SES index scores for the block groups are presented grouped into quartiles in Table 3.3.

Table 3.2
Distribution of SES Index Scores: Block-Group Data (N= 207,805)

SES Index Score	N	%	Cumulative %
21	1	0.0	0.0
23	1	0.0	0.0
25	1	0.0	0.0
26	2	0.0	0.0
27	5	0.0	0.0
28	9	0.0	0.0
29	13	0.0	0.0
30	39	0.0	0.0
31	58	0.0	0.1
32	110	0.1	0.1
33	179	0.1	0.2
34	287	0.1	0.3
35	516	0.3	0.6
36	760	0.4	1.0
37	952	0.5	1.4
38	1,392	0.7	2.0
39	1,716	0.8	2.9
40	2,260	1.1	3.9
41	2,770	1.3	5.3
42	3,457	1.7	6.9
43	4,235	2.0	9.0
44	5,243	2.5	11.5
45	6,629	3.2	14.7
46	8,058	3.9	18.6
47	10,079	4.9	23.4
48	12,053	5.8	29.2
49	14,253	6.9	36.1
50	15,738	7.6	43.7
51	16,635	8.0	51.7
52	15,852	7.6	59.3
53	14,446	7.0	66.3
54	12,496	6.0	72.3
55	10,973	5.3	77.6
56	9,355	4.5	82.1
57	7,830	3.8	85.9
58	6,338	3.1	89.0
59	5,080	2.4	91.4
60	4,223	2.0	93.4
61	3,357	1.6	95.0

(continued)

Table 3.2
Distribution of SES Index Scores: Block-Group Data (N= 207,805) (continued)

SES Index Score	N	%	Cumulative %
62	2,579	1.2	96.2
63	1,873	0.9	97.1
64	1,541	0.7	97.8
65	1,110	0.5	98.3
66	852	0.4	98.6
67	621	0.3	98.9
68	477	0.2	99.1
69	332	0.2	99.3
70	260	0.1	99.5
71	170	0.1	99.6
72	143	0.1	99.7
73	140	0.1	99.8
74	106	0.1	99.8
75	106	0.1	99.9
76	72	0.0	100.0
77	29	0.0	100.0
78	3	0.0	100.0
Total	207,805	100.0	100.0

Table 3.3
Quartile Distribution of SES Categories: Block-Group Data (N = 207,805)

SES	Category	N	%
1	(0-47)	48,772	23.5
2	(48-51)	58,679	28.2
3	(52-55)	53,767	25.9
4	(56-100)	46,597	22.4

Next, we calculated the SES index scores for the unweighted sample of 1.96 million Medicare beneficiaries we described in an earlier section of this report. This is the sample of Medicare beneficiaries on which extensive tabulations and limited multivariate modeling are to be performed. The unweighted distribution of their SES index scores is presented in Table 3.4. Note that distribution does not include 390,779 sample members who either did not have a geocode (FIPS code) or whose block group did not contain the needed Census data. The SES index scores only ran from 25 to 78.

Table 3.4
Distribution of SES Index Scores: Based on Unweighted RTI Sample of 1.96 Million Medicare Fee-for-Service Beneficiaries (N = 1,569,342)

SES Index Score	N	%	Cumulative %
25	4	0.0	0.0
26	5	0.0	0.0
27	1	0.0	0.0
28	12	0.0	0.0
29	8	0.0	0.0
30	242	0.0	0.0
31	665	0.0	0.1
32	1,092	0.1	0.1
33	2,065	0.1	0.3
34	3,785	0.2	0.5
35	4,761	0.3	0.8
36	9,288	0.6	1.4
37	13,723	0.9	2.8
38	18,758	1.2	3.5
39	22,744	1.5	4.9
40	27,185	1.7	6.7
41	31,229	2.0	8.6
42	36,960	2.4	11.0
43	41,182	2.6	13.6
44	49,166	3.1	16.8
45	59,467	3.8	20.5
46	64,802	4.1	24.7
47	79,142	5.0	29.7
48	81,865	5.2	34.9
49	94,030	6.0	40.9
50	96,156	6.1	47.1
51	105,583	6.7	53.8
52	98,188	6.3	60.0
53	93,538	6.0	66.0
54	88,403	5.6	71.6
55	76,506	4.9	76.5
56	66,203	4.2	80.7
57	56,903	3.6	84.3
58	53,307	3.4	87.7
59	40,249	2.6	90.3
60	42,205	2.7	93.0
61	29,503	1.9	94.9
62	21,694	1.4	96.3

(continued)

45

Table 3.4

Distribution of SES Index Scores: Based on Unweighted RTI Sample of 1.96 Million Medicare Fee-for-Service Beneficiaries (N = 1,569,342) (continued)

SES Index Score	N	%	Cumulative %
63	15,045	1.0	97.2
64	11,123	0.7	97.9
65	7,703	0.5	98.4
66	6,941	0.4	98.9
67	4,636	0.3	99.2
68	3,806	0.2	99.4
69	2,527	0.2	99.6
70	1,637	0.1	99.7
71	1,043	0.1	99.7
72	1,154	0.1	99.8
73	1,023	0.1	99.9
74	823	0.1	99.9
75	657	0.0	100.0
76	428	0.0	100.0
77	164	0.0	100.0
78	13	0.0	100.0
Total	1,569,342	100.0	100.0

Note: SES index scores could not be computed for 390,779 sample beneficiaries due to missing Census data or no FIPS code to link to Census data.

The distribution of SES index scores for the sample of Medicare fee-for-service beneficiaries was divided as closely as possible into quartiles. The approximate quartile distribution of the SES index scores (unweighted and weighted) is presented in Table 3.5. Note that the four categories, numbered one to four, respectively, from the category with the lowest index scores to one with highest, are the ones that we used in the tabulations and the multivariate regression analyses. One can think of the SES 1 category as representing Medicare beneficiaries in the lowest SES group, SES 4 as containing Medicare beneficiaries in the highest SES group, and those in SES 2 and SES 3 as falling in between.

We are confident that the SES index we created for this project captures the concept of SES better than any of the individual component measures because the index combines several different aspects into its composition, and the validation that follows will demonstrate that. However, the fact that nearly 20 percent of the sample of Medicare beneficiaries was not successfully geocoded and linked to the Census block group data from which the SES index was created is a definite limitation. It remains for future research on the SES index to determine whether the missing beneficiaries are a serious cause of bias. For now, having the SES index for more than 80 percent of Medicare beneficiaries provides health services researchers with opportunities for research not hitherto available.

Table 3.5

Distribution of SES Categories: Based on RTI Sample of 1.96 Million Medicare Fee-for-Service Beneficiaries (N = 1,569,342)

SES Category	Unweighted N	Unweighted %	Weighted N	Weighted %
1 (0-49)	642,181	40.9	7,967,125	29.0
2 (50-52)	299,927	19.1	6,614,863	24.1
3 (53-56)	324,650	20.7	7,214,721	26.3
4 (57-100)	302,584	19.2	5,650,911	20.6
Total	1,569,342	100.0	27,447,620	100.0

Note: SES index scores could not be computed for 390,779 beneficiaries due to missing Census data or no FIPS code to link to Census data.

3.4   Validation of the SES Measure

Before proceeding to use the four category SES measure in the tabulations and multivariate regression models, we undertook to validate the index score. To validate this measure, we needed to have a large sample similar in characteristics to the one on which we intend to run the tabulations and regression models. In addition, the sample needed to include data that we expected to be related to SES.

We used the national probability sample of Medicare beneficiary respondents to the three Medicare fee-for-service CAHPS surveys for 2002-2004 as the basis for validation of the SES measure. This was part of the sample on which we had developed the surname imputation algorithm. It happened that we had requested and received some income-related information for the respondents to those years of the survey from the Social Security Administration (SSA) for use by CMS for special analyses. We requested and received permission from CMS to use these data. The two variables from Social Security were the indexed monthly earnings (IME) that were taxed for Social Security purposes while the beneficiary was paying the Social Security tax, and the monthly benefit amount (MBA) that Social Security is currently paying beneficiaries. The former is an indicator of the beneficiary's past earned income level, while the later is a measure of the beneficiary's current benefit payments which are partly tied to past earned income level.

The first step in the validation process involved computing the SES index scores for the full validation sample. The geocode available from our previous work with these data was used to link to the Census block group data needed to calculate the SES index scores for 381,429 CAHPS Medicare fee-for-service survey respondents in the three survey years. The distribution of SES index scores was partitioned into fourths according to the groupings of scores (see categories in Table 3.5) used to create the quartiles for the analysis sample (the sample to be used in the tabulations and regression analysis for the present study). The distribution of the validation sample according to the quartile score ranges of the analytic sample is presented in Table 3.6. A comparison of the four category distribution of the validation sample to the analytic sample shows them to differ slightly, with the former composed of slightly more higher SES beneficiaries.

Table 3.6
Quartile Distribution of SES Categories: 2002-2004 CAHPS Survey Respondent Validation Sample Person-Level Data (N = 381,429)

SES	Category	%
1	(0-49)	30.6
2	(50-52)	24.5
3	(53-56)	25.5
4	(57-100)	19.4

We next computed the means of the two SSA supplied variables within each level of SES and we also cross tabulated the two SSA supplied variables with SES scores for those beneficiaries in the 2002 – 2004 CAHPS surveys for whom we were given the SSA variables. For the cross tabulations, both the SES and SSA variables were partitioned into four levels.

The top half of Table 3.7 shows the mean value of the indexed monthly earnings (IME) that were taxed for Social Security purposes within each of the SES quartile categories. Clearly the mean IMEs increased as the SES level rose, and the test of significance of mean differences across the four levels of SES is highly significant. The distribution of beneficiaries across the four categories of SES according to the four categories of their IME is also presented in the top half of Table 3.7. The test of significance for the joint distribution is also highly significant, indicating that, proportionately more beneficiaries with lower IME are classified in lower SES categories, and proportionately more of those with higher IME are classified in higher SES categories. The lower half of Table 3.7 analyzes the relationship between the mean monthly benefit amount (MBA) and SES quartile category, as well as the cross tabulation of the four category SES measure with the four level measure of MBA. A very similar pattern to the IME is present, and both tests of significance are very highly significant as well. The mean MBA increased as the SES category went from the lowest to the highest. The cross tabulation of the two categorical measures (MBA and SES) showed the same kind of association, with proportionately more low MBA beneficiaries in the lowest SES category and proportionately more high MBA beneficiaries in the highest SES category.

In addition to the two SSA variables, we had several other variables from the CAHPS survey and one from the EDB that we believed should be related to a measure of SES. These include whether or not a beneficiary is simultaneously eligible for both Medicare and Medicaid. This EDB measure is affirmative mostly for low income beneficiaries. The remaining variables are from the CAHPS survey. They include: having additional insurance (not including Medicaid), having private insurance to cover prescription drugs, reporting health status to be fair or poor, and achieving educational status no higher than high school graduate. We have presented the distributions of the five dichotomous categorical variables for respondents to the 2002 – 2004 CAHPS surveys according to the SES index quartiles in Table 3.8.

Table 3.7
Monthly SSA Earnings/Benefits of CAHPS Medicare Fee-for-Service
Survey Respondents by SES Index Categories

Variable	SES Index Categories				N	p-value
	1 (0-49)	2 (50-52)	3 (53-56)	4 (57-100)		
Indexed Monthly Earnings (IME)						
Mean in dollars ($)	1,450.75	1,604.31	1,743.74	1,968.68	177,427	< .0001
$0-$645	28.9	24.7	22.7	20.4	177,427	< .0001
$646-$950	28.2	25.3	22.2	18.8		
$951-$1192	25.3	27.1	26.3	23.7		
$1193 or more	17.6	22.9	28.8	37.1		
Monthly Benefit Amount (MBA)						
Mean in dollars ($)	861.83	921.48	970.17	1,056.92	222,977	< .0001
$0-$762	30.3	25.5	23.3	20.1	222,977	< .0001
$763-$1513	28.6	24.7	21.7	19.4		
$1514-$2341	24.5	28.7	27.9	23.1		
$2342 or more	16.5	21.0	27.2	37.3		

Note: Disabled beneficiaries are excluded from these analyses. Significance of mean differences is tested using analyses of variance. Significance across percentages is tested using chi-square tests.

Table 3.8
Percentage of CAHPS Medicare Fee-for-Service Survey Respondents by
SES and Selected Demographic Characteristics

Variable	SES Index Categories				N	Chi-Square p-Value
	1 (0-49)	2 (50-52)	3 (53-56)	4 (57-100)		
Dually eligible (from EDB)	21.5	9.5	6.2	4.6	293,312	< .0001
Have insurance in addition to Medicare (excluding Medicaid)	62.2	78.9	84.5	87.8	292,027	< .0001
Have other insurance to cover prescription costs	50.2	56.6	61.8	65.0	281,438	< .0001
Fair or poor self-reported health	44.7	35.1	30.0	24.2	287,270	< .0001
High school graduate or less	74.7	67.5	57.6	40.0	281,332	<.0001

The tests of the joint distributions of each variable with SES are very highly significant, and the directions of the joint distributions are as expected: larger percentages of dually eligible beneficiaries, persons in poor or fair health, and persons who had no more than a high school education are in the lower SES categories, and fewer persons with other insurance (not including Medicaid) and prescription drug coverage are in the lower SES categories.

Rank-order correlation coefficients between each of the five dichotomous measures from the CAHPS sample and four level SES index as well as for between the four levels of the two SSA variables and SES are presented in Table 3.9. As with all of the previous validation measures, the direction of association is always as expected. While the magnitude of the associations is moderate, all of the associations are very highly statistically significant.

Table 3.9

Spearman Correlations of SES Index Scores with Demographic and Insurance Characteristics of CAHPS Medicare Fee-for-Service Survey Respondents

Variable	N	Correlation with SES Index
Self-reported health status	287,270	0.18***
Dual eligibility	293,312	-0.21***
Have insurance in addition to Medicare (excluding Medicaid)	292,027	0.24***
Have other insurance to cover prescription costs	281,438	0.12***
Highest grade completed	281,332	0.31***
SSA IME	177,427	0.15***
SSA MBA	222,977	0.17***

*** $p < .0001$

Note: Variable for self-reported health status is recoded, so higher values represent better health.

3.5   Association of Clinical Measures with SES Index and SSA Measures

While not a part of the planned validation analysis, at the request of the AHRQ project officer, we examined the association between the SES index we created (as well as the two SSA variables) and a series of clinical measures derived from Medicare claims. We cross tabulated several clinical measures with the SES index we created and with the two SSA measures we had for the 2002 CAHPS survey respondents. These tabulations are presented in Appendix A along with a brief discussion.

4. PRODUCING REQUESTED TABULAR ANALYSES INCORPORATING THE SES MEASURE

4.1 Overview

The second objective of this project has been to produce tabulations of Medicare beneficiary utilization that includes variables representing race/ethnicity and SES. The tabulations were to further elaborate upon tabulations that were completed for the CMS task order discussed earlier (*Health Disparities: Measuring Health Care Use and Access for Racial/Ethnic Populations*, Contract No. 500-00-0024 Task No. 8). The elaboration consisted of the addition of the newly created SES index to the tabulations. The added SES index was added as a four level categorical variable in which the numerical level of the SES variable corresponds to the quartile of the distribution of the SES index scores. Beneficiaries included in SES level 1 contained index scores that were in the first quartile (lowest values) of the SES index distribution, and beneficiaries in SES level 4 had SES index scores in the fourth quartile (highest values). Those in SES levels 2 and 3 were in the second and third quartiles with SES index scores in the next to the lowest or next to the highest quartiles, respectively. One could think of these levels as representing low, medium low, medium high, and high SES.

4.2 Tabulation Format

We have prepared approximately 1,500 tabulations covering almost 3,000 pages for this sub-task. While the measures of utilization included in the tabulations are numerous and varied, the format of the tabulations, and of the appendices in which they are included, are in much the same format. This uniformity was intended to facilitate review and use of these tabulations in subsequent analyses.

Because the tabulations are so numerous, they have been organized into separate appendices. There are four separate appendices containing tabulations. Tabulations dealing with the use of cancer screening procedures are in Appendix B. Tabulations related to secondary prevention of the complications of diabetes are contained in Appendix C. Appendix D contains tabulations involving ambulatory care sensitive conditions. The final set of tabulations in Appendix E involve hospitalizations for common discharge diagnoses and report on average length of stay in days and mean expenditures in dollars.

Each of the appendices is divided in two separately bound parts. The first part of the appendix contains weighted tabulations. The weighted tabulations represent utilization of services by the population of beneficiaries in fee-for-service Medicare during 2002, the year for which the utilization data were extracted from Medicare claims. The second part of the appendix presents the same tabulations, but they are unweighted. They are labeled as "unweighted" because they only represent the sample. The unweighted tabulations have been included so that persons using the weighted estimates can check the actual number of observations on which the estimates are based to be sure that the weighted estimates are based upon a large enough sample to be considered reliable.

The tabulations in Appendices B – E are typically presented in the same format. That format presents numbers and percentages of beneficiaries using a particular service according to race/ethnicity, SES level, gender, and age group. One exception is in Appendix B where tables may be limited to males (PSA test) or females (mammogram or Pap smear) alone. A second exception is in Appendix E, where in addition to the number and percentage of beneficiaries using the service (hospitalization), there are separate tables also presenting the mean expenditure in dollars and length of stay in days.

The numbers in the cells of the tables refer to the utilization variable. Arrayed across the top of the table is the ordinal SES measure (Total, SES level 1 (lowest), SES level 2, SES level 3, and SES level 4 (highest)). Note that the Total column only includes beneficiaries who have been assigned to one of the four SES levels. Arrayed down the left side of the table are the nominal race/ethnicity groups (Total, White, Black, Hispanic, Asian/Pacific Islander, American Indian/Alaska Native, Other, and Unknown/Missing). It should be noted that the way CMS has created the Hispanic category on the EDB is without regard to race, so it is a non-redundant category. We adopted the same approach in our algorithm for creating the improved NEWRACE variable. This means that the White, Black, Asian/Pacific Islander, American Indian/Alaska Native, and Other categories are implicitly non-Hispanic. Nested within the race/ethnicity categories are categories of gender (male, female) and age group (under 65, 65 – 74, 75 – 84, and 85 or over).

All of the tabulations present a column of numbers and a column of percentages for each SES category and the total across all four SES categories. The numbers in the columns represent the beneficiaries in the particular cell (column and row intersection) of the table who used the service being analyzed. The percentages are the result of dividing the number of beneficiaries who used the service (numerators) by the entire number of persons in the particular cell whether or not they used the service (denominators). Tables containing the denominators for the percentages in the tabulations – national and MSA, weighted and unweighted – are included in Appendix H. However, note that the denominators for the percentages in the tables in Appendix B (cancer screening) may be gender specific depending upon the utilization variable (mammogram and Pap smear include females only, PSA includes males only) and that in Appendix C for tables subsequent to Table 1 (the number of beneficiaries with diabetes), Table 1 contains the denominators for the cells because the remaining tables are based on beneficiaries identified as having diabetes.

As a courtesy to the analysts who will use the weighted tabulations, we have not suppressed any weighted estimates, regardless of how small the sample size on which they are based. However, we have appended a column containing an asterisk whenever the sample frequency in the unweighted tables on which the weighted estimate was based did not reach 50 cases, the statistical criterion that we have adopted as the minimum acceptable sample size for estimates to be considered stable or reliable. Note, that while there is only a single asterisk per cell, it applies to both estimates (percent and number, and in Appendix E to mean cost and length of stay, as well). The asterisk also appears in the unweighted tables to highlight cells containing fewer than 50 observations.

We strongly recommend to everyone using the weighted tables that they _always_ check the corresponding unweighted tables before deciding to use any numbers from the weighted tables. We definitely recommend that no weighted numbers based on fewer than 50 sample cases be cited or reported as part of this or any subsequent analysis. We do not

consider estimates in this project based on table cells of 50 or fewer sample members to be stable or reliable, and that is why we have issued this warning.

Within both the weighted and unweighted sets of tables, in all of the appendices, the tables are numbered, labeled (except for the word "unweighted"), and arranged in exactly the same way. The tables are numbered according to the letter of the appendix and start with "1" within each appendix. The numbering is complete with the weighted tables, and repeats with the unweighted. In other words, Table D-1 in the weighted part of Appendix D has a counterpart Table D-1 in the unweighted part.

The tables that are numbered only, e.g. B-2, D-6, E-12, etc., are tabulations for the entire Medicare fee-for-service population (if weighted) or sample (if unweighted) and are labeled as "National". Recall that we are also preparing similar tabulations for individual metropolitan statistical areas (MSAs). These tables always follow the tables for the national Medicare fee-for-service population (if weighted) or sample (if unweighted), but are numbered and titled differently. They are numbered with the same Appendix capital letter and number but also have a lower case letter after the number. These lower case letters run from "a" to "p". The designations "a" to "p" always correspond to the same 16 MSAs and that correspondence is presented in Table 4.1.

Table 4.1
Lower Case Table Letters and Corresponding MSAs Used in Appendix Tables

Table Letter	MSA	Table Letter	MSA
a	Los Angeles, CA[# *]	i	San Diego, CA[# *]
b	Miami, FL[#]	j	McAllen, TX[#]
c	New York, NY[# *]	k	Honolulu, HI[*]
d	San Antonio, TX[#]	l	San Francisco, CA[*]
e	Riverside, CA[#]	m	Oakland, CA[*]
f	Chicago, IL[# *]	n	San Jose, CA[*]
g	El Paso, TX[#]	o	Orange County, CA[*]
h	Houston, TX[#]	p	Washington, DC[*]

10 MSAs with largest population of Hispanics 65 years of age and over.

*10 MSAs with largest population of Asian/Pacific Islanders 65 years of age and over.

Due to their sheer volume, the tabulations included in Appendices B through E have been prepared and delivered in separately bound volumes and as separate EXCEL spreadsheet files on compact disks. Note that because some of the appendices are extremely long, we have bound Appendices B through E in two volumes each – one for the weighted tabulations and one for the unweighted. Appendix H (Denominators) has also been bound separately, but because of its small size it was not split into two volumes.

4.3   Data Sources

The tabulations in the Appendices draw on data from a number of different sources. Some of these have been mentioned in previous sections of this report. Here we intend to focus exclusively on the variables used to prepare the tabulations in the event that someone would like to repeat them.

The race/ethnicity variable is the NEWRACE variable that RTI staff developed as part of the earlier task order we have referred to several times. It should be noted that this variable was updated in the first sub-task of this task order to incorporate beneficiaries who joined Medicare between mid-2003 and October 2005, but since we were analyzing 2002 services utilization in this sub-task, we used the original NEWRACE creation based on the beneficiaries on the mid-2003 EDB.

The beneficiary gender and age group variables are based on the gender and birth date variables on the mid-2003 EDB. Age was calculated as of the end of 2002, the year for which we had claims to analyze. Age was grouped into four ordinal categories: under 65 years of age, 65 to 74, 75 to 84, and 85 years of age or over. The SES measure was discussed at length in the previous section of this report. RTI created the SES index score (and the four SES categories used in the tabulations) from block group level data representing characteristics of the residential addresses of beneficiaries extracted from Summary File 3 (SF-3) of the 2000 U.S. Census.

The largest source of data for the tabulations is Medicare claims for 2002. We abstracted the service utilization for selected health services and diagnoses for the members of the stratified probability sample of 1.96 million Medicare beneficiaries enrolled in fee-for-service Medicare for the entire calendar year of 2002. The exact data file source of the data in each table is noted at the bottom of the table.

4.4   Tabulation Contents

As we indicated earlier in this section, there are tabulations dealing with the use of cancer screening procedures, secondary prevention of the complications of diabetes, ambulatory care sensitive conditions, and hospitalizations for common discharge diagnoses based on data extracted from Medicare claims for services provided in 2002. For the tabulations on cancer screening presented in Appendix B, we examined the use of screening procedures for breast (mammography for women), cervical (Pap test for women), prostate (prostate-specific antigen or PSA test), and colorectal cancers (fecal occult blood test or FOBT, flexible sigmoidoscopy, and colonoscopy). All are covered Medicare services.

For the tabulations on secondary prevention of diabetes complications in Appendix C, we identified four services from claims filed for beneficiaries with diabetes—foot care (claims for therapeutic shoes or for a podiatry visit), eye examination (claims for diabetics with eye examinations), physiological monitoring or testing (claims for testing services for hemoglobin A1c, lipid profiling, or micro albumin for monitoring insulin needs), and instruction in self care (claims for obtaining instruction in diabetes education and self-monitoring) that are covered in the traditional fee-for-service Medicare plan.

We used claims for 15 selected diagnoses that resulted in being admitted to a hospital or observed in an emergency room during the 2002 calendar year as the basis for the set of tabulations on 15 ACSCs in Appendix D. Hospitalization for these ambulatory care-sensitive conditions (ACSCs) is useful as an indicator of inadequate access to or poor-quality of primary care (Bindman, Grumbach, Osmond, et al., 1995). Among the 15 ACSCs we examined were five chronic conditions (chronic lung disease – asthma and chronic obstructive pulmonary disease combined, congestive heart failure, seizures, diabetes mellitus, and hypertension); eight acute conditions (cellulitis, dehydration, bacterial pneumonia, urinary tract infection, gastric or duodenal ulcer, hypoglycemia, hypokalemia, and ear, nose and throat infections); and two preventable conditions (influenza and malnutrition) (McCall, Harlow, and Dayhoff, 2001). Tabulations were also done for the sets of chronic, acute and preventable conditions and the diagnosis of any ACSC.

In Appendix E, we examined hospital utilization patterns among Medicare fee-for-service beneficiaries for six conditions during 2002. The conditions included heart disease, cerebrovascular disease (stroke), malignant neoplasms (cancers), diabetes, pneumonia, and fractures. In particular, we tabulated the number and proportion of persons with each of these specific diagnoses at discharge, the mean payment made per user, and the mean length of hospital stay in days.

As indicated above, the tabulations for each of these types of utilization are in separate appendices. Documentation of the programs used to create these variables in the tabulations is included in Appendix F that is bound in the report.

5. CONDUCT OF LIMITED MULTIVARIATE LOGISTIC REGRESSION ANALYSES

5.1   Introduction

Given the short project period, the small budget, and the large number of tables produced during this project, we felt it was important to attempt some initial assessment of the impact on the relationship between race/ethnicity and the use of health services of the measure of SES that we created. We believed that one way to do this efficiently was through the use of multivariate logistic regression modeling with selected utilization measures. The models were logistic because the dependent variables (measures of utilization) are all dichotomies, indicating use or no use. The models needed to be multivariate because, in addition to assessing the impact of SES on the association of racial/ethnic disparities in the use of health services covered under fee-for-service Medicare, we wanted to be able to control on beneficiary age group and gender because they are such important correlates of health services utilization and may be distributed differently across the different racial/ethnic and SES groups.

5.2   The Approach

The approach we have chosen to take with the multivariate logistic regression modeling represents a three step-approach that is easiest explained with an example. Suppose we have established in step one that there is a relationship between being Black rather than White and having a lower rate of a particular cancer screening test in the Medicare program, even after controlling for age group and gender differences between Blacks and Whites. Let us say that the difference represents a true disparity because we know that the morbidity and mortality from this kind of cancer is higher for Blacks than Whites. In addition, as we indicated, the rate of use of the screening test, which could lead to detection of this cancer at an earlier stage when it is theoretically more possible to reduce morbidity and mortality from the disease, is lower for Blacks than Whites. Then in step two of the analysis, we want to know whether rerunning the model with the inclusion of the SES measure increases, decreases, or does not change the magnitude of the disparity between Black and White utilization.

In the third step, we add the interaction of race/ethnicity and SES to the model. With this step, we want to know whether the disparity associated with race while controlling for the effects of age and gender increases, decreases, or is not affected depending on the level of the beneficiaries' SES. Finally we want to know whether any changes that occur are statistically significant and whether they are substantively meaningful in terms of reductions in disparities.

5.3   Modeling to Assess the Impact of SES

To understand the impact of SES on the association of race/ethnicity to disparities in the utilization of Medicare covered medical services while controlling for the effects of beneficiary age group and gender, we ran three different multivariate logistic regression models. In these models we analyzed seven selected utilization measures from three of the four substantive areas we included in the tabulation appendices.

The measures include three cancer screening measures (receipt in the past 12 months of: the combination of mammogram and Pap smear for women, the prostate specific antigen (PSA) test for men, and any of the three colorectal cancer screening tests for both sexes), three diabetes secondary preventive services for beneficiaries identified as having been diagnosed with diabetes (receipt in the past 12 months of: physiologic testing (hemoglobin A1c, lipid profile, or micro albumin) to monitor insulin needs, an eye exam, and instruction in self-care (diabetes education and self-monitoring)), and whether or not a beneficiary had a hospital or emergency department admission in the past 12 months with a diagnosis of any of the15 ambulatory care sensitive conditions (ACSCs) we included.

The first model was intended to impart an understanding of the relationship between a beneficiary's demographic characteristics (age, gender, and race/ethnicity) and the measure of utilization. It is at this stage that we made our initial assessment of whether a disparity in health care use exists between White beneficiaries and those of other races/ethnicities.

The first logistic model is represented as:

$$\text{logit}(\mathbf{y}_{ij} = 1 \mid race, \mathbf{x}) = \alpha + race_i + \boldsymbol{\beta}\mathbf{x}_{ij} + \varepsilon_{ij}$$

where

$race_i$ represents the effect of the ith race,

$\mathbf{y}_{ij}$ represents the response for the jth individual,

$\mathbf{x}_{ij}$ represents the covariates (age and gender where appropriate) for the jth individual,

ε_{ij} represents the residuals for the jth individual.

The second model added the SES measure to the covariates included in the first model. This second model, compared to the first, allowed us to explore how the addition of SES changed the relationships of the other covariates included in the first model.

The second logistic model is represented as:

$$\text{logit}(\mathbf{y}_{hij} = 1 \mid ses, race, \mathbf{x}) = \alpha + ses_h + race_i + \boldsymbol{\beta}\mathbf{x}_{hij} + \varepsilon_{hij}$$

where

$race_i$ represents the effect of the ith race,

ses_h represents the effect of the hth ses,

$\mathbf{y}_{hij}$ represents the response for the jth individual,

$\mathbf{x}_{hij}$ represents the covariates (age and gender where appropriate) for the jth individual,

ε_{hij} represents the residuals for the jth individual.

The third model investigated the interaction of race/ethnicity and SES. We added the interaction of SES and race/ethnicity to evaluate whether the differences in utilization among the racial/ethnic groups depended on their SES level.

The third logistic model is represented as:

$$\text{logit}(\mathbf{y}_{hij} = 1 \mid ses, race, \mathbf{x}) = \alpha + ses_h + race_i + ses * race_{hi} + \boldsymbol{\beta}\mathbf{x}_{hij} + \varepsilon_{hij}$$

where

$race_i$ represents the effect of the ith race,

ses_h represents the effect of the hth ses,

$\mathbf{y}_{hij}$ represents the response for the jth individual,

$\mathbf{x}_{hij}$ represents the covariates (age and gender where appropriate) for the jth individual,

ε_{hij} represents the residuals for the jth individual.

For all three multivariate logistic models we used SUDAAN®, a statistical analysis software package developed by RTI that is specifically designed to provide accurate analyses of weighted, cluster-correlated survey data (http://www.rti.org/sudaan/). We used the logistic regression procedure to model the probability of receiving a given treatment and we elected to use a with-replacement design because the percentage of people sampled within a given stratum was small. While we have presented the odd ratios, we have chosen to interpret the models on the basis of differences in the predicted marginals (Korn and Graubard, 1999). In logistic regression, the predicted marginal estimates the percentage or probability of beneficiaries receiving a service for a given racial/ethnic group controlling for all of the other variables in the model. The predicted marginals are equivalent to least squares means when analyzing multiple linear regression model results from a simple random sample survey.

5.4   Modeling to Establish Racial/Ethnic Health Care Disparities

From the lines in Table 5-1 for each of the services analyzed without SES in the model, we are able to establish in a preliminary way the extent to which there are racial/ethnic disparities with respect to the use of these services. The same can be done from Table 5-2 which contains the odd-ratios from the same analysis. Table 5-3 is a summary of the percentage point differences in service utilization between Whites and minorities with and without the SES measure in the model.

Looking at the age and gender adjusted predicted percentages for the first six service use measures, minorities almost always had lower utilization than Whites, suggesting disparities exist. The only exception was for receipt of instruction in diabetes self-care for which the percentage of Black diabetics getting the service equaled White diabetics. For the seventh measure, hospitalization for any ACSC, the difference in utilization indicating a disparity is reversed because a higher level of hospitalization for ACSC diagnoses is interpreted as a disparity representing poorer quality ambulatory care, i.e., hospitalization for these conditions

Table 5.1
Estimated Percent of Utilization With and Without SES Included in the Multivariate Logistic Models for Beneficiaries by Race/Ethnicity Adjusted for Gender and Age

Type of Service	SES	Race/Ethnicity				
		White[15]	Black	Hispanic	Asian/Pacific Islander	American Indian/Alaska Native
Mammogram and PAP Smear	Without SES	35%	26%*	22%*	22%*	19%*
	With SES	35	28*	24*	23*	25*
PSA	Without SES	39	30*	30*	33*	17*
	With SES	40	32*	31*	34*	25*
Any Colorectal Cancer Screening	Without SES	16	11*	10*	13*	7*
	With SES	16	12*	11*	14*	10*
Eye Exam	Without SES	62	54*	54*	58*	48*
	With SES	62	56*	58*	58*	53*
Physiologic Measures	Without SES	88	81*	82*	86*	48*
	With SES	88	82*	84*	86*	64*
Instruction in Self-Care	Without SES	54	54	47*	44*	25*
	With SES	54	52*	48*	45*	35*
Any ACSC	Without SES	7	11*	8*	5*	11*
	With SES	7	10*	8*	5*	10*

[15] White is the reference level, so all statistical tests are comparing the other race/ethnicity groups to Whites.

* Indicates p-value < 0.001

Table 5.2
Odds Ratios for Utilization With and Without SES Included in the Multivariate Logistic Models for Beneficiaries by Race/Ethnicity

Type of Service	SES	White[16]	Black	Hispanic	Asian/Pacific Islander	American Indian/Alaska Native
Mammogram and PAP Smear	Without SES	1.00	0.65	0.50	0.52	0.43
	With SES	1.00	0.71	0.58	0.53	0.59
PSA	Without SES	1.00	0.67	0.65	0.75	0.31
	With SES	1.00	0.71	0.68	0.76	0.48
Any Colorectal Cancer Screening	Without SES	1.00	0.67	0.56	0.82	0.40
	With SES	1.00	0.73	0.62	0.82	0.58
Eye Exam	Without SES	1.00	0.74	0.71	0.85	0.56
	With SES	1.00	0.79	0.86	0.84	0.70
Physiologic Measures	Without SES	1.00	0.56	0.59	0.82	0.12
	With SES	1.00	0.60	0.70	0.84	0.24
Instruction in Self-Care	Without SES	1.00	0.98	0.75	0.66	0.27
	With SES	1.00	0.92	0.77	0.67	0.44
Any ACSC	Without SES	1.00	1.60	1.12	0.66	1.55
	With SES	1.00	1.46	1.07	0.67	1.48

---

[16] White is the reference category and odds ratios are adjusted for gender and age.

Table 5.3

Summary of Adjusted Marginal Percentage Point Differences in Selected Health Services Utilization between Whites and Minority Groups With and Without SES in the Logistic Model

Type of Service	SES	Black - White	Hispanic - White	Asian/Pacific Islander - White	American Indian/Alaska Native - White
Mammogram and PAP Smear	Without SES	-9%	-13%	-13%	-16%
	With SES	-7	-11	-12	-10
PSA	Without SES	-9	-9	-6	-22
	With SES	-8	-9	-6	-15
Any Colorectal Cancer Screening	Without SES	-5	-6	-3	-9
	With SES	-4	-5	-2	-6
Eye Exam	Without SES	-8	-8	-4	-14
	With SES	-6	-4	-4	-9
Physiologic Measures	Without SES	-7	-6	-2	-40
	With SES	-6	-4	-2	-24
Instruction in Self-Care	Without SES	0	-7	-10	-29
	With SES	-2	-6	-9	-19
Any ACSC	Without SES	4	1	-2	4
	With SES	3	1	-2	3

should be avoidable with appropriate and timely ambulatory care. With this ACSC measure, there were statistically significant disparities between the rates of hospitalization for Whites and minorities. However, there was one reversal in the direction of the differences. While minorities in general had significantly higher rates of hospitalization than Whites for ACSCs, Asian/Pacific Islander beneficiaries had a lower rate that was statistically significant as well. Furthermore, the magnitude of disparities between minority beneficiaries and Whites represented by these seven utilization measures ranged from very small (e.g., Asians/Pacific Islanders) to substantial (e.g., American Indians/Alaska Natives and Hispanics).

5.5 Impact of SES on Differences in Estimated Percent Utilization

In all of the models we used to predict the utilization measures, the SES measure was statistically significant, accounting for added variance in the utilization measures. (The output of the SUDAAN® multivariate logistic regression analyses with significance test results is presented in Appendix I.) However, the increase in the amount of variance explained with the addition of the SES measure varied across the different measures of utilization. The model investigating the percentage of female beneficiaries receiving both a Pap smear and a mammogram was the least affected by the addition of SES to the model, and the model of having experienced a hospitalization for any ambulatory care sensitive condition (ACSC) was the most affected, with 1.1 percent and 22.2 percent increases in the amount of variance explained by the regression models, respectively.

The addition of SES to the models had the greatest impact on the estimated percentage of utilization for the different health care measures across race/ethnicity. The estimated percentage utilization by racial/ethnic group with SES in the logistic models controlling for age and gender (where appropriate) is also presented in Table 5.1, and the odds-ratios for the same analysis is presented in Table 5.2. Generally, when SES was added to the logistic model, the percentage of utilization for minorities increased, moving it closer to the percentage of utilization for Whites. This suggests that the racial/ethnic basis of the disparity is not as large when the effect of SES is taken into account. The results for gender and age, however, were hardly affected by the addition of SES to the model. For most measures, the percentage of utilization by gender or by age was not changed by the addition of SES to the models.

Impact of SES on Cancer Screening Use Differences. The three cancer screening measures investigated from Appendix B included the receipt during 2002 of both a mammogram and a Pap smear, a PSA test, and any of three types of colorectal cancer screening test. Across all three cancer screenings, the percentage of minority beneficiaries as compared to White beneficiaries receiving these screenings was considerably less, with American Indian/Alaska Natives almost always having the lowest utilization rates of all the minorities. For White female beneficiaries, after controlling for age, the estimated percentage receiving a mammogram and a Pap smear was 35 (Table 5.1) compared to only 19 percent for American Indian/Alaska Natives, 26 percent for Blacks, 22 percent for Asians/Pacific Islanders, and 22 percent for Hispanics. When SES was added to the model, the estimated percentage of White female beneficiaries receiving a mammogram and a Pap smear remained at 35 percent, however, the estimated percentage of minorities receiving a mammogram and a Pap smear increased. It increased to 25 percent for American Indian/Alaska Natives, 28 percent for Blacks, 23 percent for Asian/Pacific Islanders, and 24 percent for Hispanics. This represents a six percentage point reduction in the original disparity between Whites and American Indians/Alaska Natives, a two percentage point reduction for Hispanics and Blacks, and a one percentage point reduction for Asians/Pacific Islanders. The increases in their utilization after controlling for SES moved the utilization rate of mammograms and Pap smears for minorities closer to the rate of Whites. Although not completely erasing the difference in the percent of Whites and other minorities receiving both a mammogram and a Pap smear, the addition of the SES did reduce the original health care disparity.

The results of adding SES to the model were similar for the other two cancer screening measures we examined – having a PSA test, and having any of three types of colorectal cancer test. Most notable was the change in the estimated percent of male American Indians/Alaska Natives receiving a PSA test. Without SES in the model, an estimated 17 percent of male American Indians/Alaska Natives had a PSA test; 22 percentage points less than Whites. With the addition of SES to the model, the estimated percentage of American Indians/Alaska Natives receiving a PSA test increased to 25 percent while the percentage of Whites remained unchanged. This narrowed the disparity between American Indians/Alaska Natives and Whites by eight percentage points, from 22 to 14 percentage points. Similar patterns in the percentage of male beneficiaries receiving a PSA test existed for the other minority groups, but the addition of the SES variable to the model reduced the disparity between them and Whites less; two percentage points for Blacks and only one percentage point for Asians/Pacific Islanders and Hispanics.

For receipt of any of the three types of colorectal screening, the disparity between the predicted marginals of White and American Indian/Alaskan Native beneficiaries was nine percentage points, the largest in the model without SES, followed by a six percentage point disparity for Hispanics, five percentage points for Blacks, and three percentage points for Asians/Pacific Islanders. As resulted when SES was added to the model of receiving both a mammogram and a Pap smear, as well as for having a PSA test, adding SES to the model for colorectal cancer testing reduced the disparity between Whites and American Indians/Alaskan Natives to six percentage points, to five percentage points between Whites and Hispanics, to only two percentage points for Asian/Pacific Islanders, and to four percentage points between Whites and Blacks.

Impact of SES on Secondary Diabetes Prevention Services Use Differences. The diabetes utilization rates were calculated among beneficiaries with diagnosed diabetes; approximately 13 percent of Medicare beneficiaries were identified as having diabetes. Among Medicare beneficiaries diagnosed with diabetes, those receiving physiologic measures (hemoglobin A1c, lipid profile, or micro albumin) had the highest percentage of utilization among the three measures modeled; eye exam and instruction in self-care were the other two measures modeled. An estimated 88 percent of White beneficiaries diagnosed with diabetes received physiologic measurement services compared to 81 percent of Blacks, 86 percent of Asians/Pacific Islanders, 82 percent of Hispanics, and only 48 percent of American Indians/Alaska Natives. When controlling for SES, the estimated percentage of American Indian/Alaska Native beneficiaries with diabetes receiving physiologic measures increased by 16 percentage points, thereby narrowing the difference between Whites and American Indians/Alaska Natives from 40 percentage points to 24 percentage points. The estimated adjusted marginal percentage of the other minority groups receiving physiologic measures also increased, thus drawing them closer to the estimated White rate (which did not change), although not as dramatically as for American Indians/Alaska Natives. Without controlling for SES, the percent of Blacks and Hispanics receiving physiologic measures is seven and six percentage points less than Whites, respectively. However, when we controlled for SES in the model, the difference from Whites was reduced to six and four percentage points for Blacks and Hispanics, respectively.

The difference between Whites and minority groups receiving instructions in self-care was sizeable in the first model not controlling on SES. For Asians/Pacific Islanders, this difference was ten percentage points, for Hispanics seven percentage points, and for American Indians/Alaskan Natives 29 percentage points. Controlling for SES did not change the disparity much for Asians/Pacific Islanders or Hispanics (brought them one percentage point closer to Whites), but for American Indians/Alaska Natives, the difference was reduced by ten percentage points. The results for Blacks were puzzling because without SES in the model there was no disparity with Whites, but adding SES produced a two percentage point disparity.

The final diabetes measure included in the multivariate modeling was whether or not an eye exam was received. As with all the other measures, Whites had the largest percentage receiving this service and this percentage did not change with the addition of SES to the model. Results for Hispanics and American Indians/Alaska Natives changed the most when controlling for SES. Without controlling for SES, 48 percent of American Indians/Alaska Natives and 54 percent of Hispanics compared to 62 percent of Whites received an eye exam. With SES in the model, an estimated 53 percent of American Indians/Alaska Natives and 58 percent of Hispanics received an eye exam; a four and five percentage point increase respectively for both of these minorities groups with the addition of SES to the model. The percentage of Blacks receiving this service also increased when controlling for SES, but only by two percentage points. The percentage of Asians/Pacific Islanders receiving this service did not change by having SES in the model.

Impact of SES on Differences in Hospitalization for Any Ambulatory Care Sensitive Condition. This measure behaved differently than the cancer screening and diabetes preventive services utilization measures. Asian/Pacific Islanders had the lowest percentage of ACSC hospitalizations, with Whites next, and with Blacks, Hispanics, and American Indian/Alaskan Natives having the most. The changes resulting from the addition of the SES measure were very small for this measure. Blacks and American Indians/Alaskan Natives were the only groups with any change and the percentage of both of them having a hospitalization for an ACSC dropped by one percentage point, moving them closer to the rate of Whites.

5.6   Impact of Adding an SES-Race/Ethnicity Interaction Term to the Model.

To fully investigate how race/ethnicity and SES work in explaining the variance of these health care utilization measures, we ran a third logistic model that included the interaction of race/ethnicity and SES. This model enabled us to investigate whether changes in the utilization of services differed by race/ethnicity depending on the level of the beneficiary's SES. In general, as SES level increased so did the rate of utilization, regardless of race/ethnicity. The amount of improvement in utilization, nonetheless, did to some extent depend on the beneficiary's race/ethnicity. In general, White beneficiaries seem to be deriving most of the overall improvement in amount of service use as SES status increased, while Hispanics benefited the least amount. The estimated percentages of service use by SES level and race/ethnicity with age and gender controlled are presented in Table 5.4.

Table 5.4
Percentage of Beneficiaries Receiving Selected Services by Race/Ethnicity and SES Level

| Race/Ethnicity | SES Level | Cancer Screening Services | | | Diabetes Secondary Prevention Services | | | ACSC |
		PSA	Mammogram and Pap Smear	Any Colorectal Cancer Screening	Eye Exam	Physiologic Measures	Instruction in Self-Care	Any ACSC
Total	1	35%	30%	13%	57%	85%	56%	9%
	2	37	34	15	61	87	54	8
	3	40	35	17	63	88	52	7
	4	42	36	18	64	89	49	6
White	1	35	31	14	57	87	57	8
	2	38	35	15	62	88	56	7
	3	42	37	17	65	90	53	7
	4	44	38	19	66	90	49	6
Black	1	30	26	11	54	80	55	11
	2	33	27	12	55	82	52	10
	3	32	27	12	56	82	50	10
	4	33	28	13	58	84	50	9
Hispanic	1	30	22	10	57	83	49	9
	2	31	25	11	56	84	48	8
	3	31	26	11	57	85	47	7
	4	29	23	11	58	84	48	6
Asian/Pacific Islander	1	34	19	13	56	85	47	5
	2	32	23	13	57	86	44	5
	3	34	24	14	59	87	42	5
	4	35	25	15	61	88	43	4
American Indian/Alaska Native	1	22	22	9	52	60	34	12
	2	24	25	10	53	67	38	11
	3	24	25	10	52	66	35	10
	4	28	28	12	54	68	35	9

Impact of SES-Race/Ethnicity Interaction on Cancer Screening Use Differences. For all three cancer screening measures, as SES status increased from the lowest level to the highest, so did the utilization for White beneficiaries; nine percentage points for males receiving a PSA test, seven percentage points for the percent of females receiving both a mammogram and a Pap smear, and five percentage points for beneficiaries receiving a colorectal exam. Although, improvements in the rate of service use for the minority groups existed, the improvement was, with only a few exceptions, much less than for White beneficiaries. This was especially true for the Hispanics, whose increase in service use from low SES to high SES did not exceed one percentage points for any of the three cancer screening measures.

For colorectal cancer screening, the amount of improvement as SES status increased did not exceed two percentage points for Blacks or Asians/Pacific Islanders and it was only three percentage points for American Indian/Alaska Natives, but for Whites there was a five percentage point increase from the lowest to the highest SES level. Likewise, the percent of male Hispanic and male Asian/Pacific Islander beneficiaries receiving a PSA test changed only one percent from lowest to highest SES level. However, for Black and American Indian/Alaska Native males, the percentage receiving a PSA test increased three and six percentage points, respectively, as SES level increased. Yet, for White males there was a nine percentage point increase from lowest to highest SES level.

The combined results for mammogram and Pap smear were slightly different than the other two cancer screening measures. White female beneficiaries had the highest utilization and Asians/Pacific Islanders had the lowest utilization, across all levels of SES, yet, the rate of increase was similar for the two groups (seven and six percentage point increases for Whites and Asian/Pacific Islanders, respectively). American Indians/Alaska Natives had a six percentage point change also. Utilization went relatively unchanged for Blacks, and Hispanics as SES level increased from lowest to highest.

Impact of SES-Race/Ethnicity Interaction on Secondary Diabetes Preventive Service Use Differences. Among the three diabetes health care utilization measures, eye exam demonstrated the most interesting interaction. At the lowest SES level, receipt of an eye exam differed across race/ethnicity groups by five percentage points, with White and Hispanic beneficiaries having the highest (57 percent) and American Indian/Alaska Native beneficiaries, the lowest (52 percent). As SES level increased, the percentage of White beneficiaries receiving an eye exam increased at a much greater rate than for the minority groups; nine percentage points for Whites compared to five percentage points for Asian/Pacific Islanders, four percentage points for Blacks, two percentage points for American Indians/Alaskan Natives, and only one percentage point for Hispanics.

The percentage of minority beneficiaries receiving the physiologic measure services changed moderately going from low SES to high SES. Asians/Pacific Islanders and Whites experienced a three percentage point increase, while Blacks had a four percentage point increase, from low to high SES. Hispanics and American Indians/Alaska Natives were the exceptions. Hispanics only saw a one percentage point increase while American Indians/Alaska Natives changed eight percentage points from low to high SES.

The one unexpected result we obtained among the diabetes use measures was associated with the receipt of instruction on self care. We found that as the level of SES increased, the percentage of beneficiaries receiving instruction in self-care decreased. This decrease occurred across all race/ethnicity groups, but most notably for White, Black, and Asian/Pacific Islander beneficiaries. At the lowest SES level more White beneficiaries received instructions in self-care (57 percent) than any other group (34 percent for American Indians/Alaskan Natives, 47 percent for Asian/Pacific Islanders, 49 percent for Hispanics, and 55 percent for Blacks). Nonetheless, the disparity between Whites and the minority groups narrowed as SES status increased. The percent of White and Black beneficiaries receiving instructions in self-care declined to 49 and 50 percent, respectively, at the highest SES level, Asians/Pacific Islanders declined to 43 percent, while for Hispanic only declined by one percent. Utilization of this service did increase slightly (one percent) among American Indians/Alaska Natives as SES level increased.

Impact of SES-Race/Ethnicity Interaction on Differences in the Use of Any ACSC. Regardless of race/ethnicity, as SES level increased, the percentage of ACSC hospitalizations for ambulatory care sensitive conditions decreased. This decreasing trend was most pronounced for Hispanics and American Indians/Alaska Natives, both of whom experienced a change of three percentage points in ACSC hospitalization from the lowest to the highest SES level. Whites and Blacks had a slightly lower decrease in the percentage of ACSC hospitalizations going from low to high SES level, two percentage points. The rate of decline for the percentage of Asian/Pacific Islander beneficiaries with ACSC hospitalizations was much smaller, declining by only one percentage point as SES level increased from the lowest to the highest level.

5.7   Conclusions from the Modeling

The conclusions we can draw about the impact of socioeconomic status (SES) on racial/ethnic health care disparities among Medicare beneficiaries from these selected multivariate analyses are, of course, limited. We have produced tabular analyses investigating the impact of SES and race/ethnicity on 45 outcomes of interest to this task order sub-task, but we have only performed multivariate analysis on a selected seven of those. Thus, our conclusions can be little more than suggestions about what may be found upon close inspection of the tables or with multivariate analyses of more numerous utilization measures.

Across these seven analyses, it is clear that SES does impact the level of service use and therefore the disparity between the service use of White Medicare beneficiaries and those who are members of racial/ethnic minority groups. Taking into account SES does seem to reduce health care disparities, probably because the minority groups are more highly represented in the lower SES levels. However, we found that disparities between Whites and some race/ethnicity groups are more affected than others when SES is controlled. It also seems to make a difference what health service is being analyzed.

Looking at the interaction of SES and race/ethnicity is enlightening in other ways, because it suggests that for some racial/ethnic groups, the magnitude of the disparity between White and minority beneficiaries differs according to the SES level of the beneficiaries. It indicates that among some minorities, even being in the highest SES level does not make their utilization more like Whites in that same SES level. This seems to be most applicable to Hispanics and Blacks.

REFERENCES

Arday, S.L., D.R. Arday, S. Monroe, and J. Zhang. HCFA's Racial and Ethnic Data: Current Accuracy and Recent Improvements. *Health Care Financing Review.* Volume 21, Number 4, 107-116, Summer 2000.

Bindman, A.B., Grumbach, K., Osmond, D. et al. Preventable Hospitalizations and Access to Care. *Journal of the American Medical Association*, Vol. 274, No. 4, 305-311, July 26, 1995.

Bonito, A.J., Eicheldinger, C.R., Evensen, C., and Lenfestey, N. *Health Disparities: Measuring Health Care Use and Access for Racial/Ethnic Populations.* RTI Final Report for Project Number 07964.008 (in two parts plus appendices) to Centers for Medicare & Medicaid Services for Contract Number 500-00-0024, Task No. 8. Research Triangle Park, North Carolina, 2005.

Braveman, P.A., Cubbin, C., Egerter. S., Chideya. S., Marchi. K.S., Metzler. M., Posner. S. Socioeconomic status in health research: one size does not fit all. *JAMA*. 2005 Dec 14;294(22):2879-88.

Eggers, P.W. and L. G. Greenberg. Racial Differences in Hospitalization Rates among Aged Medicare Beneficiaries, 1998. *Health Care Financing Review.* Volume 21, Number 4, 1-15, Summer 2000.

Falkenstein, M.R., and Word, D.L.: *The Asian and Pacific Islander Surname List: As Developed from Census 2000.* Bureau of the Census, December 2002.

Kawachi I, Berkman L, eds. *Neighborhoods and Health*. New York: Oxford University Press; 2003.

Korn, E. L., and B. I. Graubard. 1999. *Analysis of Health Surveys*. New York: Wiley.

Krieger N, Chen JT, Waterman PD, Rehkopf DH, Subramanian SV. Painting a truer picture of US socioeconomic and racial/ethnic health inequalities: the Public Health Disparities Geocoding Project. *Am J Public Health*. 2005 Feb;95(2):312-23.

Krieger N, Chen JT, Waterman PD, Soobader MJ, Subramanian SV, Carson R. Choosing area based socioeconomic measures to monitor social inequalities in low birth weight and childhood lead poisoning: The Public Health Disparities Geocoding Project (US). *J Epidemiol Community Health*. 2003a Mar;57(3):186-99.

Krieger N, Chen JT, Waterman PD, Soobader MJ, Subramanian SV, Carson R. Geocoding and monitoring of US socioeconomic inequalities in mortality and cancer incidence: does the choice of area-based measure and geographic level matter?: the Public Health Disparities Geocoding Project. *Am J Epidemiol*. 2002a Sep 1;156(5):471 82. Review.

Krieger N, Waterman P, Chen JT, Soobader MJ, Subramanian SV, Carson R. Zip code caveat: bias due to spatiotemporal mismatches between zip codes and US census-defined geographic areas--the Public Health Disparities Geocoding Project. *Am J Public Health*. 2002b Jul;92(7):1100-2.

Krieger N, Waterman PD, Chen JT, Soobader MJ, Subramanian SV. Monitoring socioeconomic inequalities in sexually transmitted infections, tuberculosis, and violence: geocoding and choice of area-based socioeconomic measures--the public health disparities geocoding project (US). *Public Health Rep.* 2003b May-Jun;118(3):240-60.

Krieger N, Waterman P, Lemieux K, Zierler S, Hogan JW. On the wrong side of the tracts? Evaluating the accuracy of geocoding in public health research. *Am J Public Health.* 2001 Jul;91(7):1114-6.

Landis, J.R., and Koch, G.G. The measurement of observer agreement for categorical data. *Biometrics, 33*, pp. 159 - 174, 1977.

Lauderdale, D.S. and J. Goldberg. The Expanded Racial and Ethnic Codes in the Medicare Data Files: Their Completeness of Coverage and Accuracy. *American Journal of Public Health*, Volume 86, Number 5, 712-716, May1996.

McCall, N., Harlow, J., and Dayhoff, D. Rates of Hospitalization for Ambulatory Care Sensitive Conditions in the Medicare+Choice Population. *Health Care Financing Review*, Vol. 22, No. 3, 127-145, Spring 2001.

Scott, CG. Identifying the race or ethnicity of SSI recipients. *Social Security Bulletin,* Vol. 62, No. 4, 9-20, 1999.

Subramanian SV, Chen JT, Rehkopf DH, Waterman PD, Krieger N. Racial disparities in context: a multilevel analysis of neighborhood variations in poverty and excess mortality among black populations in Massachusetts. Am J Public Health. 2005 Feb;95(2):260-5. Erratum in: *Am J Public Health.* 2005 Mar;95(3):375.

U.S. Department of Health and Human Services. *Healthy People 2010: Understanding and Improving Health.* 2nd Edition. Washington, D.C.: U.S. Government Printing Office, November, 2000.

Waldo, DR. Accuracy and Bias of Race/Ethnicity Codes in the Medicare Enrollment Database. *Health Care Financing Review,* Winter 2004-2005/Volume 26, Number 2.

Word, D.L., and Perkins, R.C. Jr.: *Building a Spanish Surname List for the 1990's – A New Approach to an Old Problem.* Bureau of the Census, Population Division Technical Working Paper No. 13, March 1996. Available at: http://www.census.gov/population/documentation/twpno13.pdf.

www.ingramcontent.com/pod-product-compliance
Lightning Source LLC
Chambersburg PA
CBHW081411280526
45788CB00009B/3058